ON-SITE EMERGENCY RESPONSE

PLANNING GUIDE

For Office, Manufacturing, and Industrial Operations

SECOND EDITION

RICHARD T. VULPITTA, CUSA, NSA

DEAN R. LARSON, PHD, CEM

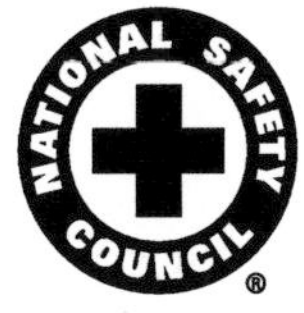

1121 Spring Lake Drive
Itasca, IL 60143-3201

Senior Director, Publishing: Suzanne Powills
Editor: Phyllis Crittenden
Text, Cover, and Interior Design and Composition: Jennifer Villarreal
Cover Images: ©2011 Thinkstock, Stock.xchng

Disclaimer

Although the information and recommendations contained in this publication have been compiled from sources believed to be reliable, the National Safety Council makes no guarantee as to, and assumes no responsibility for, the correctness, sufficiency, or completeness of such information or recommendations. Other or additional safety measures may be required under particular circumstances.

Library of Congress Cataloging-in-Publication Data
Vulpitta, Richard T.
  The on-site emergency response planning guide for office, manufacturing, & industrial operations / Richard T. Vulpitta, Dean R. Larson. -- 2nd ed.
       p. ; cm.
  Includes bibliographical references.
  ISBN 978-0-87912-311-6
  1. Emergency management. I. Larson, Dean R. II. National Safety Council. III. Title.
  [DNLM: 1. Disaster Planning--organization & administration--United States--Handbooks. 2. Industry--United States--Handbooks. 3. Safety Management--organization & administration--United States--Handbooks. HD 49]
  HV551.2.V85 2011
  363.34'525--dc22
                                                                                                            2011014198

D0511   Product Number: 12219-0000

CONTENTS

Preface viii

About the Authors ix

How to Use This Guide x

SECTION I: Basics of Emergency Planning 1

Why Prepare 2

Six Phases of Emergency and Disaster Management 2

Emergency or Disaster? 3

    Lines of Defense: Local, State, and Federal. 4

Roles of Government 4

    Steps for Establishing On-Site Emergency Response Plans 5

    Purpose of Planning. 5

    Planning Effectiveness 5

    Elements of Emergency Planning. 6

    Hazard Assessment. 6

    Toxic Materials and Material Safety Data Sheets (MSDS) 7

    Reviewing the Plan with Employees 8

    Chain of Command. 8

Lines of Communication and Warning Alarm Systems. 8

    Reporting Emergencies 9

    Assembly Areas and Command Centers. 10

    Accounting for Personnel. 10

    Disabled Employees. 10

    Special Response Teams 10

Training. 11

Additional Planning Considerations. 11

    Vehicle Fleets 11

    Personal Protective Equipment (PPE). 12

    Respiratory Protection 12

    Confined Space Entry 13

    Medical Assistance 14

    Security 14

    News Media. 14

    Business Records 15

    Response Agreements. 15

Insurance Review 15
References 15
Appendix A: Standards That Refer to 1910.38(a) Emergency Action Plan (EAP) 16
Appendix B: Standards That Refer to 1910.38(b) Fire Prevention Plan (FPP) 17
Appendix C: What Is a State OSHA Program? 18

[Note to Emergency Planner: The following Section is designed to help you build a customized On-Site Emergency Response Plan for your operation.]

SECTION II: Developing the On-Site Emergency Response Plan 19

SECTION II-A: Setting Up Your Plan 20
Purpose of Planning - Share With All Employees 22
Emergency Response Strategy and Chain of Command 22
Emergency Response Strategy 24
Initial Notification 24
Assessment 25
Command and Coordination 25
Protective Action 25
Parallel Action 26
Community Emergency Response Principles 26
Types of Disasters and Concerns About Toxic Releases 26
Emergency Management System 26
Emergency Director Overview of Duties 26
Off-Site Disaster Duties 27
Off-Site Disaster Field Response 27
Emergency Contact and Notification List 28

SECTION II-B: Building and Establishing Your Plan 32
Hazard Analysis Process 33
Hazard Analysis Form 34
Hazard Assessment Response/Recovery Information 36
Communications 38
Guidelines for Reporting Emergencies (Work or Home) 38
Fire Detection, Fire Fighting, and Alarm Systems 39
Evacuation Alarms and Fire Detection Systems 39
Use of Fire Extinguishers 41
Establishing Chain of Command and Response Roles 42
Emergency Director 44
Assistant Emergency Director 44
Emergency Coordinator 45
Assistant Emergency Coordinator 45
Stairwell Monitors 46
Searchers 47
Special Response Teams 48
Emergency Response Duties for All Employees 48

[Note to Emergency Planner: For the following Section, remember not every variable can be covered in a written procedure. Use common sense as required. The primary goal is to protect life.]

SECTION II-C: Action Plans—Site-Specific Emergency Response Plans. 50

General Evacuation Procedures. 51
    Responsibilities of All Facility Personnel. 51
    Use of Evacuation Procedure 51
    Summary of Duties for Employees. 52
Alternate Site Relocation Plan 52
Weather-Related Emergencies 52
    NOAA and General Communications. 52
    Extreme Heat Emergencies. 53
    Extreme Cold Emergencies 54
    Lightning, Thunderstorms, and Electrical Contacts 54
    Floods 56
    Hurricanes/Typhoons. 59
    Tornadoes 61
    Tsunamis (Tidal Waves) 64
Bomb Threat Procedures 66
    Receiving a Threat 66
    Reporting a Threat. 66
    Deciding to Evacuate 67
    Evaluating and Documenting the Threat 67
    Deciding if the Threat Is Real. 67
    What to Do While Speaking to a Caller. 67
    Action to Take Immediately After Bomb Threat Call 68
    Letter and Parcel Bomb Recognition Points 69
    Action to Take After Receiving Suspicious Package or Encountering a Vehicle . . . .
    with Explosives 69
    Recommendations for Handling Potentially Contaminated Mail. 71
Medical Emergency Response Procedures. 73
    Purpose 73
    Medical Emergency Notification 73
Outside Emergency Numbers. 74
Initial Response First Aid 74
Death Response and Notification Procedure. 75
Hazardous Materials Emergencies 76
    Courses of Action. 76
On-Site Spill or Release of Hazardous Materials. 77
    Spill. 77
    Air Release 77
    List of On-Site Hazardous Materials 77
Earthquake/Structural Failure Procedures. 78
Armed Robbery and Workplace Violence Emergency Response Procedures 79
    Preventing Robberies 79

Robbery in Progress 79
After the Robbery 79
Workplace Violence 80
Media-Related Events 81
Duties of a Company Spokesperson 81
Notifying Relatives of Injured Employees, Contractors, and/or Visitors 82
Nuclear Power Plant Radiological Event 82
Time, Shielding, and Distance 82
Alternate Site Relocation Plan 83
Preparing Your Employees for Home Emergencies 83
Home Emergency Planning Checklist 83

[Note to Emergency Planner: The purpose of the following Section is to use exercises and actual events to check the efficiency of your Emergency Preparedness Program and Emergency Plans and to ensure future effectiveness.]

SECTION III: Exercises, Templates, and Resources 87

Section III-A: Setting Exercise Performance Objectives 88
Exercise Performance Objectives (Learning from Actual Incidents) 89
Participants 89
Performance 89
Condition 89
Criterion 90
Unobservable, Required Performance 90
Competence 90
Reviewing Exercise Objectives 90
Types of Exercises or Drills 91
How to Control the Hazards in an Exercise 93
Controlling the Hazards 93
Evaluating the Exercise 96
Evaluators 96
Identifying Evaluators 96
Using the Information Learned 97

SECTION III-B: Overview/Template for Action Plan Drills/Exercises 98
Evacuation Drill/Exercise 99
Tornado Drill/Exercise 99
Bomb Threat Drill/Exercise 99
Medical Emergency Drill/Exercise 100
Hazardous Materials Emergency Drill/Exercise 100
Armed Robbery/Suspicious Person Drill/Exercise 100
Site Security Drill/Exercise 101

**SECTION III-C: Exercise Resources for Validation, Documentation, and
Improvements** **102**
Exercise Planning and Actual Event Documentation Form 103

Post-Exercise/Actual Event Meeting Critique Form 105

Coal-Fired Power Station Exercise 107

SECTION IV-A: Chain of Command, Plan Enhancements, and Safety Briefings 109

Chain of Command for Various Organizations 110

Plan Enhancements and Learning Aids. 113

Exit, Stairs, and Assembly Information. 113

Emergency Response Exam 117

Emergency Response Safety Briefings and Teaching Aids 119

Emergency Office Safety for Evacuation, Tornadoes, and Site Security. 120

Tornado Safety for Office, Field, and Home. 121

Emergency Point of Contact Overview 122

Emergency Response Procedures for Employees to Know. 123

SECTION IV-B: Emergency Planning Resources and Links 124

NFPA 1600 List of Hazards 125

OSHA Resources 127

Evacuation Planning Matrix. 127

Radiological Emergency Planning 129

Checklist for Compliance with OSHA 29 CFR 1910.38 and 1910.165. 133

Elements of an Emergency Action Plan 137

Elements of a Fire Prevention Plan. 138

FEMA Resources 139

Agency Overview. 139

Family Emergency Planning. 140

Independent Study Programs for Distant Learning. 142

Use of Social Media 142

Comprehensive Planning Guide (CPG 101) 145

Voluntary Private Sector Preparedness Accreditation and Certification Program. 145

FEMA Tribal Policy 147

References 149

SECTION IV-C: Additional Online Resources 151

Environmental Protection Agency (EPA) Links 152

EPA Databases and Tools. 152

EPA Resource Overview for Hazardous Event Response. 152

Key Links. 155

EPA Emergency Links 156

Contacts and Resources 159

Centers for Disease Control and Prevention (CDC) Links. 160

Other Useful Web Sites 165

Glossary of Terms. 167

PREFACE

Emergency Planning Is Not an Option!

Because emergency planning is not an option, the goal of this *Guide* is to provide the emergency planner with a step-by-step process for creating strategies for addressing a variety of emergency situations. The plans offered in this book, when diligently followed, will meet the objectives of emergency planning, which are to minimize the effects of emergencies on employees and to protect and preserve an organization's resources. Planning for unforeseen and potentially dangerous events is an essential component of an effective safety program.

My interest in emergency planning began as a safety supervisor assigned to write an emergency evacuation plan for a coal-fired generating station for the Northern Indiana Pubic Service Company. Over the years, I consolidated all of the company's emergency response plans into a single document for use in generating stations and district operations. The document allowed for the creation of site-specific plans, ensured regulatory compliance, and provided a standardized companywide emergency response procedure.

When I joined the National Safety Council, I used this process to revise the emergency plans for its Itasca, Illinois headquarters. On completion, the NSC recognized that this planning process could be used to save lives and resources. After witnessing the results of *not* planning for emergencies, and understanding that natural and man-made emergencies inevitably will occur, the solution was the first edition of the *On-Site Emergency Response Planning Guide*.

To assist in your planning mission, Dr. Dean Larson and I worked together to bring you the second edition of the *On-Site Emergency Response Planning Guide*. Dr. Larson, while teaching emergency management at Purdue University Calumet, used the *Guide* to teach his students to write emergency plans for companies to implement, and he was instrumental in streamlining the *Guide* from five sections to four. Because planning is everything, Dr. Larson believes the *On-Site Emergency Response Planning Guide* is the best tool for implementing an effective planning process for responding to emergencies, and his numerous contributions in all of the sections in this *Guide* reflect these feelings.

Section I is an updated review of the government's role, principles of emergency planning, and often overlooked preplanning considerations based on actual events and best practices. This information will better prepare the emergency planner to begin the planning process outlined in Section II.

Section II is redesigned to accelerate plan development. Expanded and new Action Plans are set in template format for the emergency planner to easily implement. I thank the National Weather Service, and especially George Wilcox, for providing the latest information on weather-related emergencies.

Section III focuses on validating the effectiveness of planning by performing exercises and documenting unplanned events to improve emergency response. Again, Dr. Larson, using his expertise fostered in years of military, industrial, and emergency planning experiences, developed a highly effective and understandable process for the emergency planner.

Section IV provides additional planning resources, means to convey the plan to employees, and links to provide you further insight and resources. I thank Dr. Larson for his contributions to all of sections in this edition of the *Guide*.

Retired NASA flight director, manager, and motivational speaker Eugene "Gene" Kranz coined the phrase "failure is not an option" when he was mission control director during the Apollo 13 crisis. Gene's credo, which is also the title of his inspirational book, brought out the best in the engineers working together to save three astronauts after their spacecraft was crippled from an explosion, and it helped carry the team through the crisis. The *On-Site Emergency Response Planning Guide* provides emergency planners with the resources needed to complete their planning mission because *emergency planning is not an option!*

Richard Vulpitta
CUSA, NSA
April 2011

ABOUT THE AUTHORS

Richard T. Vulpitta, CUSA, NSA

Rick Vulpitta has more than 25 years of utility safety experience. His leadership positions include president of the Illinois Safety Council, utilities division manager at the National Safety Council, and safety supervisor at the Northern Indiana Pubic Service Company. In the field of emergency field deployment, and as a volunteer, he served four years as director of emergency operations for the North West Indiana American Red Cross. Vulpitta is presently a regional safety manager at Comcast and has spoken nationally on the topics of emergency response planning and safety. Vulpitta is a certified utility safety administrator through the National Safety Council and is a designated national safety administrator.

Dean R. Larson, PhD, CEM

Dr. Dean Larson is experienced in military, industrial, federal, and international programs designed to prevent, mitigate against, prepare for, respond to, and recover from the unexpected. He holds a PhD, master's, and bachelor's degrees from Purdue University as well as a master's degree from the Naval Postgraduate School. Captain Larson retired from the U.S. Navy after 30 years of regular and reserve service and retired from United States Steel Corporation after serving as safety & IH manager for Gary Works, Gary Indiana. Larson is the U.S. head of delegation chair of the U.S Technical Advisory to ISO/TC 223 on *Societal Security*, a principal member of the National Fire Protection Association (NFPA) 1600 Technical Committee, and commissioner on the Indiana Emergency Response Commission (IERC) and the Certified Emergency Manager (CEM®) Commission. He is certified as an emergency manager, safety professional, performance technologist, and lead business continuity auditor. In 1999, Larson served as co-manager of the Department of Energy (DOE) POPEYE exercise, and he leads the development of the first International Organization for Standardization (ISO) standard on exercises and testing.

How to Use This *Guide*

- Completely review all Sections of the *Guide*
- Complete a hazard assessment of your facility (See Section II-B for hazard assessment instructions and a hazard assessment form).
- Complete Sections II-A, II-B, and II-C.
- Communicate your plan and train your employees to use it.
- Practice your plan.
- Review and update your plan as needed.

A companion CD is included with this *Guide* that is designed to assist you in writing and customizing an emergency response plan for your facility. Follow the prompts in this *Guide* and fill out the forms provided on the CD to create a customized plan that can be saved and updated as needed.

SECTION I
BASICS OF EMERGENCY PLANNING

In Section I, you will learn the need for emergency planning, the roles of government, and factors an emergency planner needs to consider for developing an emergency plan:

- Why Prepare?

- Six Phases of Emergency and Disaster Management

- Emergency or Disaster?

- Roles of Government

- Steps for Establishing On-Site Emergency Response Plans

- Lines of Communication and Warning Alarm Systems

- Training

- References

- Appendix A: Do You Need an OSHA Emergency Response Plan?

- Appendix B: Do You Need a Fire Prevention Plan?

- Appendix C: What Is a State OSHA Program?

WHY PREPARE?

In a 10-minute span of time, two people will be killed and 740 will suffer an injury severe enough to require consultation with a medical professional.* On average, 15 unintentional-injury deaths and about 4,440 medically consulted injuries occur every hour during the year. Unintentional injuries are the leading cause of death for all persons between 1 and 44 years old, and for all age groups they are the fifth leading cause of death (NSC, *Injury Facts*®, 2011, pp. 10, 31). The emergency planner must acknowledge the potential for every type of human emergency and natural disaster and establish plans to lessen the event's effects. Emergency planning is an extension of an effective workplace safety and health program.

SIX PHASES OF EMERGENCY AND DISASTER MANAGEMENT

Emergency and disaster management is an ongoing process of planning for and responding effectively to the occurrence of an unplanned event. The process consists of the following six phases:

1. Prevention—eliminating a hazard or stopping an emergency event in progress
2. Mitigation—steps taken to lessen the effects (consequences) of an emergency or disaster event
3. Preparedness—planning for an emergency or disaster event
4. Response—the planned response to an emergency or disaster event
5. Recovery—the process of returning to normal operations
6. Continuity—policies, plans, and procedures put in place to ensure the continued delivery of critical functions throughout response and recovery

When these six phases are used together, they lessen disaster and emergency spillover effects that can disrupt local operations and quality of life. For example, the following spillover effects can result from a river overflowing its banks due to heavy rains:

- Normal lines of communication are lost.

- The floodwaters disrupt transportation and utility services to the area.

- Several of the residents and workers fleeing the rising water are injured or killed.

- Factories and residences are damaged or destroyed.

- Hazardous materials are released.

- Local medical facilities are quickly rendered inadequate.

- Looting occurs.

- Local resources are quickly exhausted and state and federal assistance is required to mitigate the effects for a return to normal operations.

---

*Starting with the 2011 Edition of *Injury Facts*, the National Safety Council adopted the definition of medically consulted injuries to replace disabling injuries.

Advanced planning and recognition of the spillover effects of a disaster can lessen the impact on local residents and businesses. For example, a community can become "flood-smart" by taking the following steps:

- Establish an early warning system for residents and businesses in the potential floodplain.

- Clearly mark evacuation routes along higher-ground areas to aid movement of residents to safety.

- Keep the storage of hazardous materials by local industry to a minimum.

- Practice for disasters at medical facilities.

- Enact building codes that prevent new companies from locating in areas of potential floodwaters.

- Inform the public not to drive or walk onto roads that are flooded.

EMERGENCY OR DISASTER?

To understand emergency and disaster management, you need to understand their similarities and differences.

Similarities

- They begin as unexpected occurrences.

- They produce negative effects.

- They have to be dealt with immediately.

- The responses have similar goals.

Differences

- They have different resources available.

- They have different methods of response.

- They have different scopes or impacts.

The goals of *emergency and disaster response* are similar:

- To protect and save people.

- To protect property.

- To resume normal activities.

The differences between *emergencies* and *disasters* lie in the methods of response. Responses to emergencies use local resources. Responses to disasters can initially be local, but when local resources become exhausted, outside responders and/or resources are needed. Once these outside resources successfully overcome the disaster, normal activities are resumed.

Another difference between the two is scope or impact. Disasters tend to affect all normal activities in a large geographic area. Emergencies are more contained, disrupting normal activities in a particular community or a single facility.

Lines of Defense: Local, State, and Federal

In emergency planning/disaster preparedness, governmental activities are divided among local, state, and federal entities. Laws outline the responsibilities of each governmental level during an emergency or disaster event. The responsibilities are broader at the state and federal levels. The responsibilities of each level are as follows:

- local
  - responsible for local planning
  - responsible for initial response
- state
  - plans for statewide disasters
  - allocates reserve resources
- tribal
  - plans for emergencies and disasters that impact tribal lands
  - identifies / allocates tribal reserve resources
- federal
  - responsible for national disasters
  - backs up state resources

Local town/city or county police, fire, and medical personnel who respond to human and natural emergencies are the first line of defense. If the local responding agencies require additional assistance, the county where the event took place provides the resources and personnel. When the emergency exhausts the resources of that county, the county's governing body requests assistance from the governor of that state. If state resources are exhausted or inadequate, the governor can request disaster relief in writing from the president of the United States. The president authorizes various federal agencies to assist. One of these agencies is the Federal Emergency Management Agency (FEMA). At this time, FEMA would become involved with recovery efforts. Besides the goal of mitigating the event, the local, state, and federal agencies share the goal of uninterrupted governmental activities.

ROLES OF GOVERNMENT

Each level of government has characteristic resources it can bring to bear on emergency management. The resources of each level can be summarized as follows:

- Federal: legal authorities, fiscal resources, research, technical information and services, specialized personnel
- State: legal authorities, administrative skills, conduit between local and federal levels

- Tribal: legal authorities, can have local knowledge of the situation, personnel, proximity to both event and resources

- Local: direct motivation, knowledge of the situation, personnel, proximity to both event and resources

STEPS FOR ESTABLISHING ON-SITE EMERGENCY RESPONSE PLANS

If the objective is to achieve an effective workplace emergency procedure for a facility, an effective workplace safety and health program must be in place. The importance of an effective workplace safety and health program cannot be overstressed. Benefits from such a program include increased productivity, improved employee morale, reduced absenteeism and illness, and reduced workers' compensation rates. Businesses without safety and health plans should address this issue. The National Safety Council, a not-for-profit, non-governmental organization, is one of several organizations that can assist in the development of safety and health guidelines and the training of personnel. However, sometimes injuries occur in spite of efforts to prevent them. For this reason, planning for anticipated or likely emergencies is necessary to minimize employee injury and property damage.

Facilities that have a successful safety and health program almost always have an effective emergency procedure already in place. For these companies, the *On-Site Emergency Response Planning Guide* can be used to review, update, and revise the existing emergency response programs or, because of its format, it can be used to convey the plan to employees.

Purpose of Planning

The purpose of planning is to outline the basic steps needed to prepare to handle emergencies in the workplace. These emergencies may include accidental releases of toxic gases, chemical spills, fires, explosions, personal injury, or natural disasters. Emergency response plans are not intended to be all-inclusive, but rather to provide guidelines to the people who use the plan for overcoming emergencies.

Planning Effectiveness

The effectiveness of response during emergencies depends on the amount of planning and training performed. Management must show its support of facility safety programs and the importance of emergency planning. If management is not interested in employee protection and minimizing property loss, little can be done to promote a safe workplace. It is therefore management's responsibility to see that a program is instituted and that it is frequently reviewed and updated. The input and support of all employees must be obtained to ensure an effective program. The emergency response plan should be developed as a team effort involving all levels of management and employees.

Elements of Emergency Planning

The plan should be comprehensive enough to deal with all types of emergencies and clearly written to be easily understood. Minimal elements of the plan should include the following:

- List emergency escape procedures and emergency escape route assignments.
- Provide procedures to be followed by employees who remain to perform (or shut down) critical plant operations before they evacuate.
- Provide procedures to account for all employees after a completed evacuation.
- Conduct training and practice with the proper equipment for employees who are called on to perform special duties, such as rescue, medical duties, hazardous response, fire fighting, etc.
- Provide the preferred means for reporting fire, medical, and other emergencies that occur on-site.
- Provide a chain of command listing names or regular job titles of persons or departments who are responsible for emergency decision-making and response actions.
- Identify hazards and determine the likelihood of their occurrence (hazard assessment).
- Develop various emergency responses for the types of emergencies likely to occur.
- Conduct training and practice for employees.
- Update the plan at least annually and communicate revisions as needed to employees.

See Section II-C, Site-Specific Action Plans.

Hazard Assessment

Emergency response plans are based on the identified potential emergencies that can reasonably be expected to occur at a particular workplace. To create such plans, first identify all potential emergencies. Examples of potential emergencies addressed in this Guide include fire, chemical release, critical injury, etc. Then conduct a hazard assessment (also known as a risk evaluation or hazard audit) on each historical or current potential emergency. Use outside sources to assess hazards. Contact your insurance carrier; state, county, and local emergency planning agencies; and National Weather Service for a history of hazardous events.

Have an assessment team of personnel familiar with the operations of the site review each hazard assessment. For example, a review team for an office building would include a maintenance engineer, office supervisor, and safety manager. A power plant review team would include these and an operations supervisor. The assessment team analyzes on-site emergencies by determining "what if" and "how bad will it be" if this event occurs. Each event must be evaluated objectively by considering frequency, intensity, and duration.

The emergency planners also need to determine if emergencies in nearby businesses might present hazards. In many communities, the local fire department is the conduit of information to the community. You may consider contacting them on what local operations pose a hazard that would need a response plan in place and what information is available to assist in dealing with this off-site hazard.

Lines of transportation may also be considered a source of potential hazard. For example, if a truck crash on a nearby highway releases a chemical vapor into the air, employers in the area may need to take action to protect their employees. Therefore, it is necessary when performing a hazard assessment to consider the potential for an off-site emergency to affect your place of operation.

Hazard assessments include the following components:

- critical equipment list—If critical equipment fails and causes an emergency, determine the potential consequences of various failure scenarios. Determine the minimum personnel needed to monitor and operate the equipment in the event of an emergency.
- site utilities list—Determine suppliers, entry points, and shutoffs for on-site utilities such as air-handling systems (HVAC), electric, gas, water, and communications. Determine the need for and extent of backup systems.
- natural disasters—Determine the potential effects of natural disasters, such as tornadoes, blizzards, ice storms, tidal waves, hurricanes, earthquakes, mud slides, floods, and/or fires.
- man-made disturbances—Determine the possible effects of a bomb threat, arson, riot, vapor release, chemical release, terrorist attack, and structural failures.
- transportation lines—Determine if shipping, rail, air, or highway emergency events may have a spillover effect on a facility.
- toxic materials and/or raw materials—Determine if a potential hazard exists on-site.
- other site spillovers—Determine the effects of potential spillover emergency events from other facilities.

See Section II-A, for Hazard Assessment information and completion forms.

Toxic Materials and Material Safety Data Sheets (MSDS)

Toxic materials released into the environment can cause unsafe conditions. If an emergency planner needs information on the chemicals at a facility for which plans are being written, he can contact the manufacturer or supplier for a material safety data sheet (MSDS) on the material or substance. An MSDS includes the following sections:

- manufacturer's information
- hazard ingredients
- physical chemicals
- fire and explosive hazards data
- reactivity data
- health hazard data
- precautions for safe handling and use
- control measures

The hazard information from the MSDS can be of great assistance in planning and evaluating a company's ability to respond to a chemical emergency. As previously mentioned, risk management plans and other chemical release information from facilities in the surrounding community are available through the EPA or the local emergency planning committee.

Reviewing the Plan with Employees

Based on the hazard assessment, plans need to be written for the identified potential emergency situations. All employees must be told what actions they are to take in various emergency situations that may occur in the workplace. For emergency evacuation, floor plans or workplace maps clearly showing the emergency escape routes and safe or refuge areas need to be included in the plan. These also need to be posted throughout your facility. (See Section IV, for sample maps of evacuation exits and stairways and evacuation assembly areas.)

The plan needs to be reviewed with employees when the plan is developed, whenever the employees' responsibilities under the plan change, and whenever the plan is changed. A copy should be kept where employees can refer to it at convenient times. As a best practice, the employer should provide each employee with a copy of the plan during initial training. Plans need to be reviewed and explained to all new employees when they are hired. The elements of emergency planning and templates for various emergencies are included in this Guide and are available on a companion CD.

Chain of Command

A chain of command should be established to minimize confusion so employees will have no doubt about who has authority for making decisions. Responsible individuals should be selected to coordinate the work of the emergency response team. In larger organizations, there may be a facility coordinator in charge of all facility operations, department coordinators who supervise particular department operations, and others. Because of the importance of these functions, adequate backup must be arranged so that trained personnel are always available. (See Emergency Response Roles for employees in Section II.)

The duties and responsibilities of those at the top of the chain of command should include the following:

- assessing the situation and determining whether an emergency exists that requires activating the emergency procedures

- directing all efforts in the area, including evacuating personnel and minimizing property loss

- ensuring that outside emergency services, such as medical aid and local fire departments, are called in when necessary

- directing the shutdown of plant operations when necessary

LINES OF COMMUNICATION AND WARNING ALARM SYSTEMS

Lines of communications between outside emergency response agencies and the on-site employees are the most critical part of an emergency response plan and one of the first to fail. Emergency communications need to include primary and backup equipment, such as portable phones, alarm systems, amateur radio systems, public address systems, or portable radio units, for notifying employees of the emergency and for contacting local outside emergency agencies.

The warning alarm system is a method of communication needed to alert employees about evacuation or to take other action as required in the plan. Alarms should be audible or seen by all people in the facility. These systems need to have an auxiliary power supply in the event electricity is affected. The alarm should be distinctive and recognizable as a signal to evacuate the work area or perform actions designated under the emergency action plan. A backup portable air-horn system may have to be considered in the event the main alarm is inoperable.

Another consideration is that the alarm system may not be heard in all areas of a facility or by employees with physical impairments. As a best practice, repeat the alarm several times, followed by public address announcements. Also, facilities should install visual alarm systems for the hearing impaired. Another best practice is to have pre-appointed search teams of two enter areas where alarms may not be heard to alert employees of the emergency response action to take.

Reporting Emergencies

The employer needs to explain to each employee the means for reporting emergencies, such as manual pull-box alarms, public address systems, or calling a certain in-house telephone number. Emergency phone numbers should be posted on or near telephones or in other conspicuous locations. It may be necessary to notify other key personnel, such as the plant manager or physician, during off-duty hours. An updated written list of these numbers needs to be available to key personnel at all times (Figure 1).

EMERGENCY REPORTING GUIDELINES

All emergencies (fire, bomb threat, medical or any other) shall be reported immediately to the Operator at Extension ___________. The operator will call for appropriate outside assistance.

- When reporting an emergency by phone, start by giving your name, department, extension number, and exact location. Report the emergency event as clearly and accurately as possible. Remember, in any situation, it is important to remain calm.

- The Receptionist/Dispatcher may need additional information. Stay on the line; do not hang up first. The Receptionist/Dispatcher will either tell you to hang up or will hang up on you.

- If it is fire-related, describe the equipment involved, smoke, fire and size. After your call to the Receptionist/Dispatcher, only attempt to extinguish a fire when your personal safety is not in jeopardy.

SITE-SPECIFIC EVACUATION ALARM INFORMATION

THE ALARM SYSTEM FOR THIS LOCATION IS: ___________________________________

IT IS LOCATED: ____

____

Figure 1. Effective communication is the most important single element of emergency response and the first critical element to be lost during an emergency. All employees need to be instructed on how to report emergencies.

Assembly Areas and Command Centers

During a major emergency involving a fire or explosion, it may be necessary to evacuate offices and manufacturing areas. To account for all employees, a prearranged assembly area communicated to employees in advance is essential. This is known as the primary assembly area. In the event the primary assembly area is unavailable, it is necessary to have an alternate assembly area to which employees can report. Designated assembly areas for employees need to be in areas that outside emergency response service agencies will not be using. The assembly site becomes a focal point for incoming and outgoing communications. The facility person designated as being in charge will make the assembly site the command center. The command center serves as an area to meet with the responding outside emergency agencies and to account for evacuees.

Accounting for Personnel

In the event of an evacuation, management will need to know when all personnel have been accounted for. This can be difficult during shift changes or if contractors are on-site. A responsible person should be appointed to account for personnel and to provide that information to the designated person in charge of the site during an emergency. The names of those believed to be missing will be forwarded to the facility person in charge, who will forward this information to the proper responding outside emergency agencies.

Disabled Employees

If your facility has employees who may be physically or mentally limited, assign at least two employees to assist each person during any emergency. These assignments need to be made prior to an emergency. Those assigned would assist in an appropriate fashion in the event of any emergency. For additional information on accommodations for disabled employees, see the National Organization on Disability: www.nod.org.

Special Response Teams

In emergencies, special response teams may become the first line of defense for a facility. The type and extent of the emergency will depend on the facility operations. The response will vary according to the type of process, the material handled, the number of employees, and the availability of outside resources. Special response teams may need training in the following procedures:

- use of various types of fire extinguishers
- first aid, including cardiopulmonary resuscitation (CPR)
- emergency shutdown procedures
- confined space, overhead structure, or underwater rescue
- chemical spill-control procedures
- use of self-contained breathing apparatus (SCBA) and other respirators
- incipient and advanced-stage firefighting

Special response teams need to be trained in the types of emergency actions to be performed. In certain instances they may need to be certified. Specific training requirements are stated in the OSHA standards. Employees need to be trained and have the opportunity to practice their skills. The members of these special teams may need to be provided with special equipment, and they must be physically able to perform their specialized duties.

TRAINING

Training is important for the effectiveness of an emergency plan. Before implementing an emergency action plan, a sufficient number of key people must be trained to assist in administering the key elements of the plan. All other employees need to be trained on how to respond to each type of emergency. This will enable employees to know what actions are required. Employees also need to understand that they must use common sense when responding in any emergency situation. In addition to specialized training for key people, other employees should be trained in the following:

- evacuation plans and routes

- when to avoid elevator use

- alarm identifications

- reporting emergency conditions

- shutdown procedure responses for identified emergencies

- the use of common sense when necessary

- smoke inhalation dangers and how to crawl under smoke to escape to safety

- how to check closed doors for the presence of heat and smoke

The emergency response procedures should be written in concise terms and made available to all personnel. When should training occur? Training programs need to be held as follows:

- initially when the plan is developed, then annually

- for all new employees

- when new equipment, materials, or processes are introduced

- when procedures have been updated or revised

- when a drill or an actual emergency event determines that an improvement needs to be communicated to employees

(See Section IV for training aids in the form of safety benefits.)

ADDITIONAL PLANNING CONSIDERATIONS

Vehicle Fleets

If your organization has a fleet of vehicles the following suggestions are based on actual occurrences. If your vehicle fleet is garaged on-site and the drivers are the only ones who have the keys, have a spare set for each vehicle at the site. In the event vehicles must be relocated during an emergency, your drivers might not be available or able to respond. The extra set of keys on-site and planning for others to respond will protect your fleet. Over several thousand vehicles are lost every year while parked in areas that were never to be flooded, or in the area of fire because the keys to move them were not available.

Personal Protective Equipment (PPE)

Effective personal protection is essential for anyone who may be exposed to potentially hazardous substances. In emergency situations employees can be exposed to a variety of hazardous circumstances, including the following:

- chemical splashes or contact with toxic materials
- falling objects and flying particles
- unknown atmospheres that may contain toxic gases, vapors, mists, or inadequate oxygen to sustain life
- fire and electrical hazards

It is extremely important that employees be adequately protected in these situations.

Emergency planners should consider whether personal protective equipment (PPE) is required to safely respond to an incident. Planners should specify what PPE is to be used, where it is to be located, who is responsible for maintaining it, and how it is to be used in an emergency. If PPE is specified for escape, drills should incorporate the wearing of PPE during evacuation. (See the following section on respiratory protection for OSHA standard minimum compliance requirements that must be met before assigning or using PPE.)

Some of the safety equipment that can be used includes the following:

- safety glasses, goggles, or face shields for eye protection
- hard hats and safety shoes for head and foot protection
- proper respirators for breathing protection
- whole-body coverings, gloves, hoods, and boots for body protection from chemicals
- body protection for abnormal environmental conditions, such as extreme temperatures

The equipment selected must meet criteria contained in the OSHA standards.

The choice of protective equipment is not a simple matter. Therefore, consult with health and safety professionals before making any purchases. Manufacturers and distributors of health and safety products may be able to answer questions if they have enough information about the potential hazards involved.

Respiratory Protection

Consult with professionals when providing adequate respiratory protection.

Respiratory protection is necessary for toxic atmospheres of dusts, mists, gases, or vapors and for oxygen-deficient atmospheres. Self-contained breathing apparatus (SCBA) offers the best protection to employees involved in controlling emergency situations. SCBA should have a minimum rating oxygen supply of 30 minutes. Conditions that require use of a SCBA include the following:

- leaking cylinders or containers
- smoke from chemical fires
- chemical spills that indicate high potential for exposure to toxic substances
- atmospheres with unknown contaminants
- atmospheres with unknown contaminant concentrations
- confined spaces or oxygen-deficient atmospheres

The OSHA standard minimum compliance requirements must be met before assigning or using respiratory equipment. These requirements are as follows:

- written respiratory protection program with worksite-specific procedures
- proper respiratory protection selection procedures
- medical evaluations of employees required to use respirators
- employee training of respiratory hazards in routine and emergency situations
- employee fit testing for tight-fitting respirators
- routine use and emergency use procedures
- respiratory cleaning, disinfecting, storage, inspection, repairing, discarding, and other maintenance procedures
- atmosphere-supplying respirator procedures to ensure adequate air quality, quantity, and flow of breathing air
- employee training of proper use and limitations of respirators
- program evaluating procedures
- air sampling

For additional respiratory protection information, go to the NIOSH Web site at www.cdc.gov/niosh/homepage.html.

Confined Space Entry

Detailed plans need to be in place prior to entry into any confined spaces. All on-site confined spaces need to be identified. Personnel are never to enter a confined space unless the components of the confined space entry program have been followed and appropriate permits have been completed. These include atmospheric testing of oxygen, upper and lower explosive level limits, and toxins.

Confined spaces can contain a variety of hazards, including toxic gases, explosive atmospheres, and oxygen deficiency. Other hazards that also must be considered are electrical hazards, hazards created by mixers or impellers, and exhaust fumes from combustion engines. Hazards need to be controlled, deactivated, locked-out, or removed. Communications between all workers within and outside the confined space need to be maintained. Lifelines are to be unobstructed and untangled.

In the event of an emergency situation, those rescue procedures written and practiced in advance need to be activated.

Medical Assistance

In a medical emergency, time is a crucial factor in minimizing injuries. Most small businesses do not have a formal medical program, but they are required to have the following medical and first-aid services reasonably available:

- In the absence of an infirmary, clinic, or hospital in close proximity (6 to 10 minutes) to the workplace that can be used for treatment of all injured employees, the employer must ensure that a person or persons adequately trained to render first aid are present on-site.

- The employer must ensure the ready availability of medical personnel for advice and consultation on matters of employee health. This does not mean health care must be provided, but rather, if health problems develop in the workplace, medical help will be available to resolve them.

- The employer must survey the medical facilities near the place of business and make arrangements to handle routine and emergency cases. A written emergency medical procedure needs to be included as part of an emergency response plan.

- If the business is located far from medical facilities, at least one and preferably more employees on each shift must be adequately trained to render first aid. The National Safety Council, American Heart Association, local safety councils, fire departments, and others may be contacted to provide this training.

- First-aid supplies need to be provided for emergency use. This equipment should be ordered through consultation with a physician familiar with the particular workplace hazards.

- Area ambulance services need to be surveyed to determine response time, emergency handling capabilities, and hospital locations. Ambulance services need to be familiarized with a facility's location and access routes in advance.

Security

During an emergency, it is often necessary to secure the area to prevent unauthorized access and to control the event. An off-limits area must be established. Access by emergency vehicles should not be impeded. Mechanical gates should be secured in an upright position to facilitate the movement of emergency vehicles. Security needs to guide emergency personnel to the area where they are needed. All entries and exits need to be documented by time. If there is an electronic entry system, it can supply information on the employees who are on-site. (Also note that if there is an electronic entry system, a power failure coupled with the emergency can freeze the entry system. It may be necessary for security to know how to manually activate entry operations.)

News Media

If the emergency is newsworthy, representatives from the press also will be present. Establish an area for the press so they can be briefed on a regular basis as facts are established. This keeps the press together and allows for the accurate release of information. Establish in advance the management official who will oversee the role of company spokesperson. When approached by members of the press, all employees at the site should refer the reporter to the official company spokesperson.

Business Records

Certain records, essential to the survival of your business, need to be protected. Such essential information may include accounting files, equipment information, procedures, product specifications, insurance information, financial information, legal documents, employees' home phone numbers, their relatives to be notified in case of emergency, customers, vendors, suppliers, contractors, and so on. The on-site emergency planning committee will need to determine what information is critical to facility and business operations.

The on-site emergency planning committee will also need to consider how to protect daily business transactions and daily computer information that is generated as well as any critical information. This may require that information be protected in a secure location within the facility or in off-site storage. The planning committee will also need to consider protection of the daily or weekly backup of computer-generated critical transactions or information ensuring the survival of a business or facility.

Response Agreements

Any type of emergency mutual-aid agreement needs to be in writing and detailed as to services provided. These agreements need to be in place with suppliers and providers of specialized services critical to a facility during a disaster or an emergency.

Insurance Review

Review with your insurance carrier the type of coverage you now have, what actually would be covered (building, contents, computer systems, injuries, etc.), and the dollar amounts of the coverage of your facility and its contents. It is also important to have your insurance carrier identify the emergency or disaster the policy will or will not cover.

REFERENCES

Emergency Management Institute National Training Center. *Introduction to Emergency Management.*

U.S. Department of Labor—Occupational Safety and Health Administration Various sources on information for preparing for workplace emergencies.

National Safety Council. *Injury Facts 2011 Edition.* Itasca, IL: National Safety Council, 2011, pp. 10, 31.

Section II of this Guide contains templates that will assist in developing a specific on-site emergency plan for a facility by completing the information through a step-by-step process. To further assist, all sections are reproduced on a companion CD. Follow the instructions and prompts when inputting information. The text may also be modified for your specific planning needs.

APPENDIX A

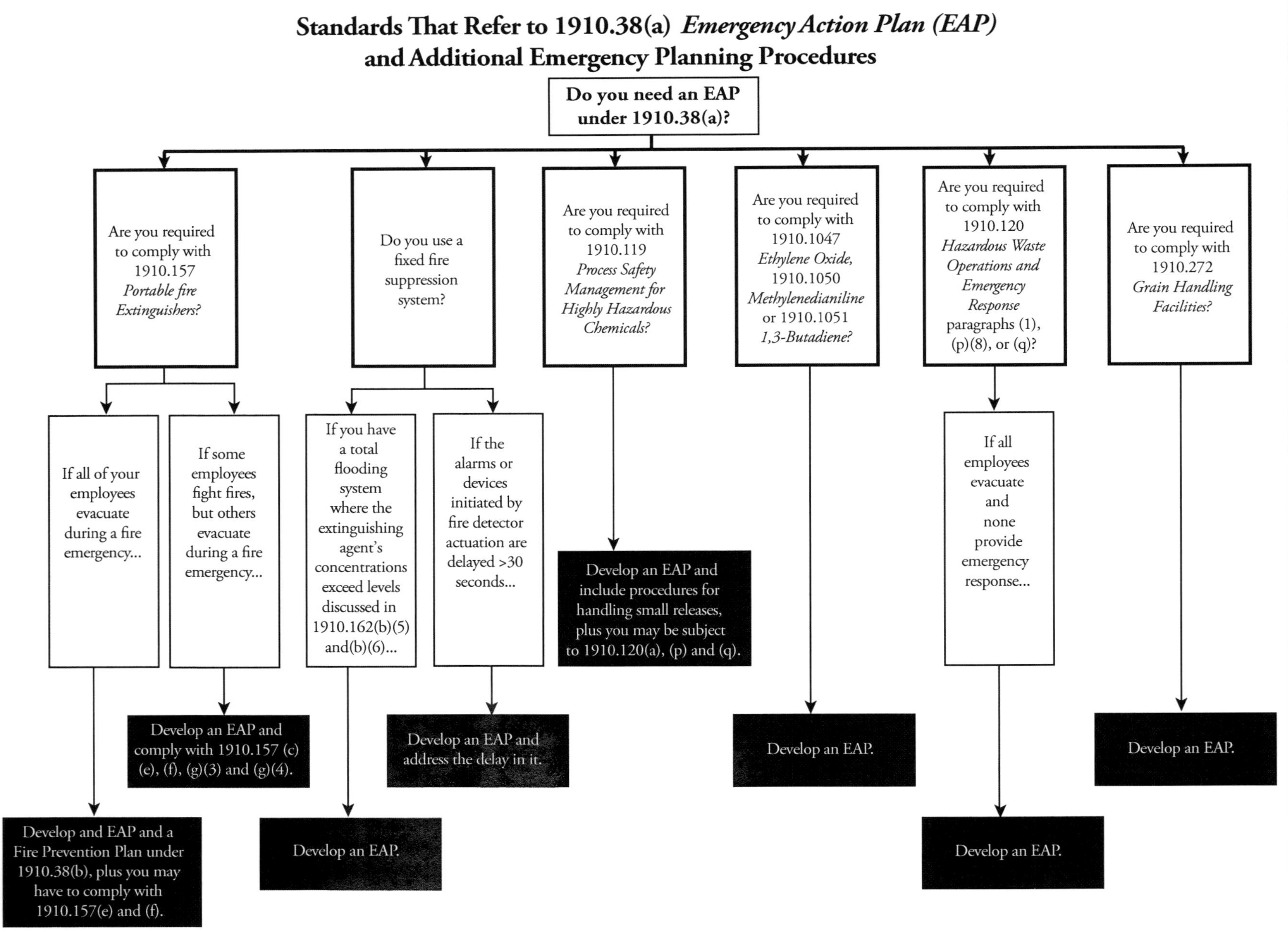

Standards That Refer to 1910.38(a) Emergency Action Plan (EAP) and Additional Emergency Planning Procedures

Do you need an EAP under 1910.38(a)?

Are you required to comply with 1910.157 Portable fire Extinguishers?
If all of your employees evacuate during a fire emergency...
Develop and EAP and a Fire Prevention Plan under 1910.38(b), plus you may have to comply with 1910.157(e) and (f).
If some employees fight fires, but others evacuate during a fire emergency...
Develop an EAP and comply with 1910.157 (c) (e), (f), (g)(3) and (g)(4).

Do you use a fixed fire suppression system?
If you have a total flooding system where the extinguishing agent's concentrations exceed levels discussed in 1910.162(b)(5) and(b)(6)...
Develop an EAP.
If the alarms or devices initiated by fire detector actuation are delayed >30 seconds...
Develop an EAP and address the delay in it.

Are you required to comply with 1910.119 Process Safety Management for Highly Hazardous Chemicals?
Develop an EAP and include procedures for handling small releases, plus you may be subject to 1910.120(a), (p) and (q).

Are you required to comply with 1910.1047 Ethylene Oxide, 1910.1050 Methylenedianiline or 1910.1051 1,3-Butadiene?
Develop an EAP.

Are you required to comply with 1910.120 Hazardous Waste Operations and Emergency Response paragraphs (1), (p)(8), or (q)?
If all employees evacuate and none provide emergency response...
Develop an EAP.

Are you required to comply with 1910.272 Grain Handling Facilities?
Develop an EAP.

APPENDIX B

Standards That Refer to 1910.38(b) *Fire Prevention Plan (FPP)* and Additional Emergency Planning Procedures

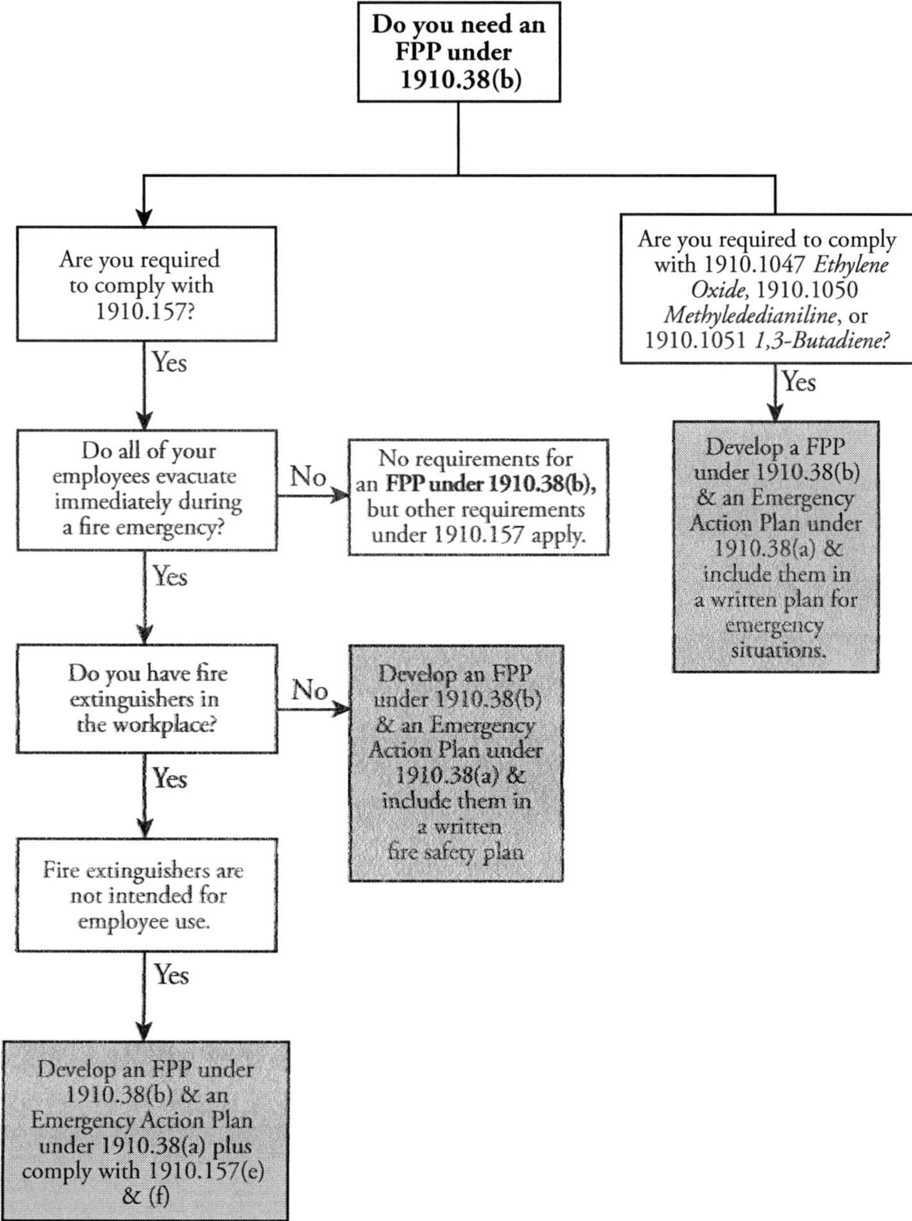

APPENDIX C

What is a State OSHA Program?

Section 18 of the Occupational Safety and Health Act of 1970 encourages States to develop and operate their own job safety and health programs. OSHA approves and monitors State plans and provides up to 50 percent of an approved plan's operating costs.

There are currently 23 States and jurisdictions operating complete State plans (covering both the private sector and State and local government employees) and three — Connecticut, New Jersey and New York — which cover public employees only. (Eight other States were approved at one time but subsequently withdrew their programs).

Alaska	Maryland	Oregon	Washington
Arizona	Michigan	Puerto Rico	Wyoming
California	Minnesota	South Carolina	
Connecticut	Nevada	Tennessee	
Hawaii	New Mexico	Utah	
Indiana	New Jersey	Vermont	
Iowa	New York	Virgin Islands	
Kentucky	North Carolina	Virginia	

(Please note that the Connecticut, New Jersey and New York plans cover public sector employment only) [Current as of: October 29, 2002]

SECTION II
DEVELOPING THE ON-SITE EMERGENCY RESPONSE PLAN

[To the emergency planner: You will want to write your plan starting in this section. Section II is divided into three parts—A, B, and C. Each section is designed to build a specific part of your facility's plan.]

Read the entire Guide before completing the information requested in this section. When you have completed the requested information for each area, Section II will become your complete plan. Delete all prompts and instructions addressed to the emergency planner.

In Section II-A, you will learn to:

- understand emergency principles
- develop a notification system
- assign key emergency responding duties to employees
- conduct hazard assessments

In Section II-B, you will identify alarm and fire-fighting systems and make them part of your plan.

In Section II-C, you will customize the pre-written "Action Plans" for your facility's needs. Action Plans have been included for man-made and natural events.

SECTION II–A
SETTING UP YOUR PLAN

The general purpose of developing on-site emergency response procedures is to anticipate emergencies and mitigate the potential for loss of life and property. Instituting appropriate response procedures minimizes the impact of an emergency, and keeping these procedures simple will help employees remember how to respond. A chain of command during an emergency will be established for your employees with defined titles and duties. The concepts and principles of on-site emergency planning will be reviewed and will be come part of your plan.

- Purpose of Planning
- Emergency Response Strategy and Chain of Command
    - Initial Notification
    - Assessment
    - Command and Coordination
    - Protective Action
    - Parallel Action
- Community Emergency Response Principles
    - Interaction with Outside Agencies
    - Community Emergency Response Principles
- Types of Disasters and Concerns
- Emergency Management System
    - Off-Site Disaster Duties (Toxic Releases and Exposures)
    - Off-Site Disaster Response
- Emergency Contact and Notification List

[To the emergency planner: When you have completed all of the requested information for each area of Section II, delete the prompts that provide instructions and address the emergency planner.]

[To the emergency planner: This is your title page. Complete the requested information]

This Emergency Plan is for

____

Street Adress

City / State / Zip

Site phone: (XXX) XXX-XXXX

Remember not every variable can be covered in a written procedure.
Use common sense as required. The primary goal is to protect life.

If there are any questions regarding this procedure contact: _______________________

At: _________________________________

PURPOSE OF PLANNING – SHARE WITH ALL EMPLOYEES

1. To Protect Life – our first goal is to protect employees

2. To Protect Property – our second goal is to protect property and the environment so we may continue to have a place to conduct business

3. To Return to an Operating Level (this may not be a full or normal operations level)

Establishing emergency procedures for the protection of facility employees is an important component of the facility's safety program. This Guide consolidates and standardizes the various procedures written for this facility. This document has been developed by:

who is the facility's designated Emergency Planner(s).

[Add name of your Emergency Planner(s) above.]

EMERGENCY RESPONSE STRATEGY AND CHAIN OF COMMAND

The following gives an overview of an emergency response strategy and covers the typical chain of command in emergency management. The five-point emergency response strategy is:

1. initial notification
2. assessment
3. command and coordination
4. protective action
5. parallel action

The general purpose of developing on-site emergency response procedures is to anticipate emergencies and mitigate the potential for loss of life and property. Instituting appropriate response procedures will minimize the impact of an emergency. All employees must understand their responsibilities and those of their co-workers in the event of an emergency.

The Emergency Response Strategy and Chain of Command Overview outlines the response strategy and command chain for dealing with emergencies.

[To the Emergency Planner: Read the entire Guide before completing the information requested in this section. When you have completed the requested information for each area, delete the prompts addressed to the emergency planner]

The Emergency Operations Center is where all emergencies are first reported during normal working hours. It is located where there is an employee dedicated to receiving calls during normal hours of operation.

1. Initial Notification is received at our site at the Emergency Operations Center, located:

____.

During non-emergencies this functions as a ___________________________________.

[To the Emergency Planner: The position most likely to be assigned this responsibility could be the: 1) Receptionist 2) Security Guards 3) Administrative Assistant 4) Executive Secretary, etc. Insert the appropriate title and position into the above request, then delete this prompt]

2. This person has the authority to contact outside agencies to respond to this site for the reported emergency.
3. The next step is to notify the Emergency Director who will assess the situation.
4. The appropriate Action Plan is then activated to protect life. Protecting property is discussed in Section II-C.
5. Parallel action involves placing a call to outside agencies that have greater emergency resources to overcome an emergency. For example, if someone is having a heart attack, you would call for an ambulance.
6. Employees should respond as they have been trained. Response roles are detailed in Section II-B.

The chain of command is overviewed to highlight the roles of those involved in responding.

[To the Emergency Planner: Customize these positions and titles for your facility as desired or as required for your operation.]

The Emergency Director is the highest-ranking emergency official and will direct the response activities during an emergency.

[To the Emergency Planner: Include the statement below as representative of your operation, otherwise delete the next paragraph]

Our organization has a number of sites, and it is impractical for the Emergency Director to cover all sites at the same time. At these sites an "Emergency Coordinator" will be the highest-ranking emergency official to direct the response activities during an emergency.

- At least one Assistant Emergency Director should be designated in the event the primary Emergency Director is unavailable.

- An Emergency Coordinator needs to be designated for each department or business unit at the facility. An Assistant Emergency Coordinator also is designated for each department or business unit at the facility. The Alternate or Assistant Emergency Coordinator assists the Emergency Coordinator.

- The Stairwell Monitors should be those employees closest to stairway fire doors (in multi-story buildings).

- The Searchers are employees who are pre-assigned by each department or business unit who work in pairs to locate employees who may not have heard the emergency announcement.

The Special Response Team Members are employees who have received specific training to respond to reasonably anticipated specific emergencies such as a chemical spill or medical emergency.

Emergency Response Strategy

The emergency response strategy is a five-point strategy outlining the essential points of any response plan. The five points are initial notification, assessment, command and coordination, protective action, and parallel action. Complete the information for your facility in the spaces provided below.

Initial Notification

It is the responsibility of all employees to report immediately all incidents or conditions that pose a threat to life or property.

[To the Emergency Planner: The position most likely to be assigned this responsibility could be the: 1) Receptionist 2) Security Guards 3) Administrative Assistant 4) Executive Secretary, etc. Insert appropriate title and position into the above request, then delete this prompt]

Call the Emergency Operations Center at: ____________________ext. _______ during working hours.

During normal operations, this area functions as the: ____

During off-hour emergencies, call: ____.

The person receiving the initial call will make necessary notifications regarding the reported emergency.

[To the Emergency Planner: Insert the title of the person who will assume each of the duties listed in the following sections. There may be several alternates for each position depending on the size of your facility and hours of operation. It is vital that the employee receiving the initial emergency call has immediate access to someone qualified to act as the *Emergency Director*. Similarly, depending on the number of departments and your facility layout, there may be a number of Emergency Coordinators. Your plan should specify who they are and name at least one alternate for each Emergency Coordinator.]

Emergency Director: ____.
Phone ext. (Include all ext. numbers.): ____.

Assistant Emergency Director: ____.
Phone ext. (Include all ext. numbers.): ____.

Emergency Coordinator: ____.
Phone ext.: ____.

Assistant Emergency Coordinator: ____.
Phone ext.: ____.

Emergency Coordinator: ____.
Phone ext.: ____.

Assistant Emergency Coordinator: ____.
Phone ext.: ____.

Emergency Coordinator: ______________________________________.

Phone ext.: ______________________________________.

Assistant Emergency Coordinator: ______________________________________.

Phone ext.: ______________________________________.

Emergency Coordinator: ______________________________________.

Phone ext.: ______________________________________.

Assistant Emergency Coordinator: ______________________________________.

Phone ext.: ______________________________________.

Assessment

The Emergency Director is responsible for assessing the level of an emergency. If Emergency Directors are not available or appointed, the Emergency Coordinator will take this role.

Command and Coordination

The Emergency Director is responsible for activating and coordinating the appropriate protective action plan.

The director also interfaces directly with outside emergency agencies. During an emergency or disaster, the Emergency Director may direct emergency operations from the Emergency Operations Center. The Emergency Operations Center is______________________________________.

[To the Emergency Planner: Add the locations of your facility's Emergency Operations Center (EOC) and its Backup Operations Center. The Backup should be a secure, windowless room located on the first floor.]

The Backup Operations Center, which will be used when the primary EOC cannot be used, is located at ______________________________________.

Phone ext.: ______________________________________.

Paging systems are available at ext.: ______________________________________.

[To the Emergency Planner: Add phone extensions.]

In the event that an emergency, such as fire or chemical release, could impact the Emergency Operations Center, the Emergency Director will designate an Incident Site Command Center that is outside the danger zone.

Protective Action

Protective actions are those functions that mitigate the situation to ensure the safety of personnel and property, with a planned response for an uncontrolled event.

Parallel Action

Parallel action facilitates the duties of an Emergency Director or Emergency Coordinator during an emergency response and involves on-site personnel and/or outside emergency agencies. Parallel action also refers to interaction with outside agencies and sharing of information and other resources that aid affected parties.

COMMUNITY EMERGENCY RESPONSE PRINCIPLES

This section describes the concept of the emergency management system and the way your facility Emergency Director will interact with outside agencies. If you have a multisite operation, it is impractical for the Emergency Coordinator to be at each site. In that case, the designated Emergency Coordinator will perform the duties outlined below for the Emergency Director.

Types of Disasters and Concerns About Toxic Releases

Disasters can be caused by natural or man-made events. Natural disasters include floods, tornadoes, and hurricanes. Man-made disasters include chemical releases and vehicle crashes.

Regardless of the type of disaster or where it occurs, employees must be aware that exposures to hazardous or toxic substances can occur through inhalation and skin contact. Employees should protect themselves to avoid exposure. In a disaster event contact on-site authorities for recommendations on avoiding exposure to toxic substances.

Emergency Management System

Many communities have already adopted mutual-aid agreements, as such, several community emergency agencies may respond to an emergency or a disaster to your facility. Responding agencies can include medical, police and HAZMAT teams, and fire fighters. The composition of these professionals responding needs a command structure and that is known as the Emergency Management System.

The activities of all responding outside agencies are coordinated through a central chain of command headed by one person—usually the highest ranking fire fighter at the scene. This person is known as the Incident Site Commander. The Incident Site Commander is positioned at the Incident Site Command Center, which is set up outside the area of danger. Communications are also usually headquartered at this command center. This system is also called the Incident Command System.

Emergency Director Overview of Duties

The Emergency Director commands all facility employees during an on-site emergency or disaster. He is the official representative of the facility with outside emergency agencies.

Emergency Director duties during an on-site emergency or disaster:
- Locate the Incident Site Command Center (Responding Fire Fighters Command Center)

- Introduce yourself to the Incident Site Commander (Highest Ranking Fire Fighter)

- Report roll call results to the Incident Site Commander. The roll call results will be collected by your designated Emergency Coordinators or Searchers.

- Provide information and updates to company management on response and event status.

- Contact the company's **Public Information Officer** to conduct all news releases and comments to the press.

[To the Emergency Planner: Add the title/name and contact information of your facility/site spokesman, public relations, or public information officer.]

At our various sites the Emergency Director may not be available. The "Emergency Coordinator" will be the highest-ranking emergency official to direct the response activities during an emergency and perform all duties listed above.

Off-Site Disaster Duties

Employees at the scene of an emergency or disaster outside of work must understand the Emergency Management System of responding. Remember that the nationwide Emergency Management System has been organized so that many agencies from neighboring communities and different geographic locations may respond to an emergency or disaster. Knowing how the system works is especially important if more than one emergency agency does respond and is on the scene of an emergency or disaster. When multiple agencies respond, they are directed by the Incident Site Commander.

Off-Site Disaster Field Response

The person in charge usually has the title of Incident Site Commander (see previous description of the Emergency Management System). Every disaster response is handled on a case-by-case basis. If you are at the site of an emergency (not at your place of business) before responding emergency agencies arrive, remember the following guidelines:

- Report the emergency—call 911 first. Provide details of who and what is involved.

- As an employee you are not required to provide assistance. If you do assist you do so as a volunteer.

[To the Emergency Planner: Clarify this guideline with your organization's policy. You may need to consult with your organization's legal counsel.]

- Survey the scene. If gases or chemical clouds are present, or if power lines are down, do not enter.

- Administer first aid according to training.

- Protect yourself from exposure to bloodborne pathogens. Use a barrier.

- At first opportunity, report any details to the first agency to respond.

- Contact your supervisor about the event.

[To the Emergency Planner: Complete all information for Section II-B and II-C before completing the information requested in this section. Add additional information as needed for your operation/facility.]

EMERGENCY CONTACT AND NOTIFICATION LIST

Location: ____

Phone: ________________________________ Ext: ___________

Street Address: ____

District: _______ Number of Employees Assigned: ___________

FOR BUSINESSES THAT LEASE OR RENT:

Landlord: ____

Address: ____

On-site Address: ____

Daytime Phone: ____

After-hour phone contact: ________________________________

E-mail: ____

Contact Person(s): ______________________________________

EMERGENCY REPORTING NUMBERS

On-Site: ____

Local Police: __________________ County Police: ___________

Fire: __________________ State Police: ___________________

Medical: ________________ HAZMAT Response No.: _________

Alarm Company: *INSERT NAME OF COMPANY*

Phone: ____

On-site Fire Equipment: *INSERT NAME OF COMPANY*

Phone: ____

On-site Fire Protection System: *INSERT NAME OF COMPANY*

Phone: ____

Site Facilities or Building Services: *INSERT NAME*

Phone: ____

Company spokesman, public relations, or public information officer: *INSERT NAME*

Phone: ____

Key Department Emergency Personnel/Duties (See Section III for details)

Manager: ________________________Wk/Hm Phone: _________

Emergency Coordinator: ______________________ Phone: ______

*Emergency Coordinator: ______________________ Phone: ______

**Emergency Coordinator: _____________________ Phone: ______

*To be updated as needed by Emergency Coordinator. To be forwarded twice each year to the Emergency Planning Committee.
**Designates alternates or assistants. Attach additional information if needed.

Department Searchers (Male/Female): _______________________________________

Unoccupied Areas to Search: ____

Stairwell Monitors Stairwell Exit/Alternate Stairs

____ Flr. __________#__________ / __________

____ Flr. __________#__________ / __________

EXIT INFORMATION

Exit # _______________ Primary for: _____________ Alternate Exit # ____________________

Exit # _______________ Primary for: _____________ Alternate Exit # ____________________

Exit # _______________ Primary for: _____________ Alternate Exit # ____________________

ASSEMBLY LOCATIONS OUTSIDE IMMEDIATE LOCATION

Primary Location: _____________________________ Alternate Location: _____________________________

WEATHER-RELATED EMERGENCY INFORMATION SAFE AREAS

____

DISASTER RECOVERY PLANNING

In the event a location cannot be reoccupied, our "Alternate Site Relocation Plan" calls for re-establishment at: ____

[To Emergency Planner: The following template is included for locations with a 24-hour operation or to be used as a form to organize additional phone information.]

EMERGENCY PHONE LISTING

Location: _____________________________ Outside Phone Lines: _____________________________

Manager: ____

Phone: (Work) _____________________ (Home) _____________________

Emergency Director: ____

Phone: (Work) _____________________ (Home) _____________________

Assistant Emergency Director: ____

Phone: (Work) _____________________ (Home) _____________________

A Shift: _____________________________ Home Phone: _____________________________

B Shift: _____________________________ Home Phone: _____________________________

C Shift: _____________________________ Home Phone: _____________________________

D Shift: _____________________________ Home Phone: _____________________________

Department	Emergency Coordinators	Backup ECOs	Searchers	Stairwell Monitors
	Ext.	Ext.	Ext.	Ext.
	Ext.	Ext.	Ext.	Ext.
	Ext.	Ext.	Ext.	Ext.
	Ext.	Ext.	Ext.	Ext.
	Ext.	Ext.	Ext.	Ext.
	Ext.	Ext.	Ext.	Ext.
	Ext.	Ext.	Ext.	Ext.
	Ext.	Ext.	Ext.	Ext.
Additional Shifts of ________				
	Ext.	Ext.	Ext.	Ext.
	Ext.	Ext.	Ext.	Ext.
	Ext.	Ext.	Ext.	Ext.
	Ext.	Ext.	Ext.	Ext.
	Ext.	Ext.	Ext.	Ext.

Additional Shifts of _______				
	Ext.	Ext.	Ext.	Ext.
	Ext.	Ext.	Ext.	Ext.
	Ext.	Ext.	Ext.	Ext.
	Ext.	Ext.	Ext.	Ext.
	Ext.	Ext.	Ext.	Ext.

[To Emergency Planner: The following contacts need to be included as part of your plan. They can be included as part of this list, in Section IV (Resource Section), or in both areas depending on your operation.]

Insurance Company: *INSERT NAME OF COMPANY*

Phone: ____

Agent's Name: *INSERT NAME* (If your site has a large event in need of immediate construction, emergency power, clean-up, etc., request your agent to the site to approve (sign or initial purchase orders) theses needed services. It should be discussed prior to an event whether the agent or a representative will perform this function.)

Phone: ____

Local and National Fire / Disaster Restoration Services: *INSERT NAME OF COMPANY(S)*

Phone: ____

Local Construction / Roofing Restoration Services: *INSERT NAME OF COMPANY(S)*

Phone: ____

[To Emergency Planner: Construction or Local Fire / Disaster Restoration Services may not be available in your area if the emergency or disaster was widespread and severe. You may need to contract these services with providers outside your local area. In either case, involve your purchasing department and get approvals in advance.]

[To the Emergency Planner: Read the entire Guide before completing the information requested in this section. When you have completed the requested information for each area, delete the prompts addressed to the emergency planner.]

- Hazard Analysis Process
  - Hazard Assessment Form
  - Hazard Assessment Response/Recovery Information
- Communications
  - Emergency Call-in Center
  - Establishing a Communication Chain
  - Reporting Emergencies during Work Hours/Nonwork Hours
  - Standardized Reporting Procedure
- Fire Detection, Fire Fighting, and Alarm Systems
  - Evacuation Alarms and Fire Detection Systems
  - Use of Fire Extinguishers
  - Establishing Chain of Command and Response Roles
    - Assigning Key Roles for Normal Working Hours
    - Assigning Key Roles for Outside Normal Work Hours
    - Responsibilities of All Employees During an Emergency

[To the Emergency Planner: Revise as needed to complete the requested information for your facility. The position most likely to be assigned this responsibility could be the: 1) Receptionist, 2) Security Guards, 3) Administrative Assistant, 4) Executive Secretary, etc.]

[To the Emergency Planner: Note that not all areas of the United States have 911 as the emergency response number. Verify that each region has 911 or insert the area's emergency response number. Verify whether a 9 or 1 must be dialed first with your telephone system to reach an emergency agency. Also verify whether your telephone prefix is local. Some large companies have area codes that are not local to their offices.]

HAZARD ANALYSIS PROCESS

[To Emergency Planner: This is a critical part of the planning process. Emergency response plans are based on the identified potential emergencies that can reasonably be expected to occur at a particular workplace. To create such plans, first identify all potential hazards. Then conduct a hazard assessment (also known as a risk evaluation or hazard audit) on each historical or current potential emergency. Use outside sources to verify hazards.]

Contact your insurance carrier; state, county, and local emergency planning agencies; and National Weather Service for a history of hazardous events.

Have an assessment team of personnel familiar with the operations of the site review each hazard assessment. (For example, a review team for an office building would include a maintenance engineer, office supervisor, and safety manager. A power plant review team would include these and an operations supervisor.) The assessment team analyzes on-site emergencies by determining "what if" and "how bad will it be" if this event occurs. Each event must be evaluated objectively by considering frequency, intensity, and duration.

The Emergency Planners also need to determine if emergencies in nearby businesses might present hazards. Lines of transportation may also have to be considered as a source of a potential hazard. For example, if a truck crash on a nearby highway releases a chemical vapor into the air, facilities in the area may need to take action to protect their employees. Therefore, it is necessary to perform a hazard assessment to determine the potential for one emergency to cascade into expanding emergencies.

[To Emergency Planner: For additional information review Hazard Assessment in Section I of this Guide.]

Hazard assessments include the following components:

- Critical equipment list—If critical equipment fails and causes an emergency, determine the potential consequences of various failure scenarios. Determine the minimum personnel needed to monitor and operate the equipment in the event of an emergency.

- Site utilities list—Determine suppliers, entry points, and shutoffs for on-site utilities such as air-handling systems (HVAC), electric, gas, water, and communications. Determine the need for and extent of backup systems.

- Natural disasters—Determine the potential effects of natural disasters, such as tornadoes, blizzards, ice storms, tidal waves, hurricanes, earthquakes, mud slides, floods, and/or fires.

- Man-made disturbances—Determine the possible effects of a bomb threat, arson, riot, vapor release, chemical release, terrorist attack, and structural failures.

- Transportation lines—Determine if shipping, rail, air, or highway emergency events may have a spillover effect on a facility.

- Toxic materials and/or raw materials—Determine if a potential hazard exists on site.

- Other site spillovers—Determine the effects of potential spillover emergency events from other facilities.

[For the Emergency Planner: When you understand theses instructions and have completed the following requested information for Hazard Assessments delete the prompts addressed to the emergency planner.]

Hazard Assessment Form

Use this form to determine the potential effects of a hazard on your operation. Identify your critical equipment/operations and the effects if they fail. Use a team approach when identifying critical operations/equipment. This assessment will be based on the likeness, duration, and impact of natural or man-made emergencies on your operation.

Contact outside sources to compile a history of the frequency and severity of past hazardous events. Use the same team to identify and build resources into your plan to overcome these hazards. Seek resources to protect critical operations or repair or replace critical equipment so your site can return to normal operations.

TYPE OF HAZARD / DISASTER / EMERGENCY: ________________________________

POTENTIAL OF OCCURRENCE – Based on historical and current information:

____

____

CONSEQUENCES CAUSED BY THE EMERGENCY: _____________________________

____

CRITICAL EQUIPMENT/OPERATION DISRUPTION: ___________________________

____

ON-SITE EQUIPMENT NEEDED TO RESPOND TO THE EMERGENCY:

____

ON-SITE SKILLS/TRAINING NEEDED TO RESPOND TO THE EMERGENCY:

____

Based on the information listed, numerically rate the potential of occurrence and consequences of the event, using the following key.

Hazard Rating Select Across	Highest Impact	Strong Impact	Limited	Rare / Minor	Total Below
Potential of Occurrence (Frequency)	Very High Value – 4	Strong Value – 3	Limited Value – 2	Rare Value – 1	
Consequences (Intensity)	Catastrophic Value – 4	Major Value – 3	Limited Value – 2	Minor Value – 1	
Duration To Emergency Planner: Revise **the Weeks and/or Days** for your site	Catastrophic **Over 2 – 3 Weeks** Value – 4	Major **1 – 2 Weeks** Value – 3	Limited **3 – 5 days** Value – 2	Minor **1 – 2 days** Value – 1	
Total Across	XXXXXXXX	XXXXXXXX	XXXX	**TOTAL**	

POTENTIAL OF OCCURRENCE RATING	
CONSEQUENCES RATING	
DURATION RATING	
TOTAL OF ALL VALUES If Consequences Rating value is 3 or 4 and the two other ratings are 3 or greater, concentrate on identifying and building resources for this hazard.	

HAZARD ASSESSMENT RESPONSE/RECOVERY INFORMATION

[To the Emergency Planner: As you perform your hazard assessments, develop a list of contacts and resources to assist in overcoming an emergency event in your operation. Below is an example of how to create a resource prior to an event. Secure the needed purchasing approvals in advance of an event. Delete this example from your final plan.]

<table>
<tr><td colspan="2">This is a completed example.
Type of Emergency: Flooding response for the training center</td></tr>
<tr><td>Company: World Wide Restoration Services
Company Land Line: (800) 555-7615
Address: 246 Clarion
City: San Diego / State: CA / Zip: 66342
Web-site: World Wide Restoration.Net</td><td>Contact Name: Brandon Jackson
Title: VP Logistics
Cell Phone: (630) 555-7614
E-mail: B_Jackson@WWRS.Net
Alternate: Sam Waters / Logistics Supv.</td></tr>
<tr><td colspan="2">Identified Emergency Issue: Flood damage clean-up and building repairs
Provider of Equipment and/or Service Provided: Specialize in all areas of flood restoration from clean-up to major repairs.</td></tr>
<tr><td colspan="2">Vendor Approval Status: Purchasing approved vendor. Standing PO on file.</td></tr>
</table>

<table>
<tr><td colspan="2">Type of Emergency:</td></tr>
<tr><td>Company:
Company Land Line:
Address:
City / State / Zip
Web-site:</td><td>Contact Name:
Office Phone:
Cell Phone:
E-mail:
Alternate:</td></tr>
<tr><td colspan="2">Identified Emergency Issue:
Provider of Equipment and / or Service Provided:</td></tr>
<tr><td colspan="2">Vendor Approval Status:</td></tr>
</table>

<table>
<tr><td colspan="2">Type of Emergency:</td></tr>
<tr><td>Company:
Company Land Line:
Address:
City / State / Zip
Web-site:</td><td>Contact Name:
Office Phone:
Cell Phone:
E-mail:
Alternate:</td></tr>
<tr><td colspan="2">Identified Emergency Issue:
Provider of Equipment and / or Service Provided:</td></tr>
<tr><td colspan="2">Vendor Approval Status:</td></tr>
</table>

Government Resources: As you perform your hazard assessments, develop a list of government contacts at the local, county, and state levels.

[To the Emergency Planner: Delermine what resources/services you will require.]

Local/City Emergency Contacts:			
Department	**Phone**	**Services**	**Notes**

[To the Emergency Planner: Delete "County" example information and replace it with your operations information for your final plan.]

County Emergency Contacts: Lake County, Indiana			
Department	**Phone**	**Services**	**Notes**
Animal Control	(219) 663-1228	Wild Animal Removal	
Health Services	(219) 663-1116	Re-occupancy Approval	
Highway Dept.	(219) 663-1222	Road Restoration	

State Emergency Contacts:			
Department	**Phone**	**Services**	**Notes**

COMMUNICATIONS

Site Emergency Call-In Center – NORMAL WORKING HOURS		
Located On Site	Name of Person / Title or Position	Phone Number

Site Emergency Call-In Center – OUTSIDE NORMAL WORKING HOURS		
Located On Site	Name of Person / Title or Position	Phone Number

If No Answer, Call for Outside Assistance. Add number(s) to reach outside line (1 or 9)			
Medical	**Fire**	**Police**	Notify On-Site Emergency Coordinator
X – 911	X – 911	X – X 911	Notify Supervisor as Required
XXX-XXXX	XXX-XXXX	XXX-XXXX	Add non-emergency number for each

Guidelines for Reporting Emergencies (Work or Home)

- To report an emergency by phone provide the following:
    - Your name, department, phone/extension number, and exact location.
    - Report the emergency as clearly and accurately as possible.
    - Remember, in any situation, it is important to remain calm.
- The inside receptionist/outside dispatcher may need additional information.
    - Stay on the line; do not hang up first.
    - When all necessary information has been given, the receptionist/dispatcher will either ask you to hang up or will end the call.

Special Emergencies

- If the emergency is medical and involves labored breathing, heavy bleeding, is heart-related or appears to be life threatening, provide that information during the call so outside responders are prepared.

[To the Emergency Planner: Provide locations of your facility alarms below.]

SITE-SPECIFIC EVACUATION ALARM INFORMATION

The evacuation alarm system for this location is: ___________________________________

It is activated by: ____

It is located: ____

It sounds like: ____

FIRE DETECTION, FIRE FIGHTING, AND ALARM SYSTEMS

Evacuation Alarms and Fire Detection Systems

[To the Emergency Planner: Complete the information requested in the following table. Revise as needed for your operation. It is advisable to have several employees on each shift be trained on operations of these systems so they can be manually activated or shut off, as needed, during an emergency]

List the names and position of employees of who are trained with each system.

SITE-SPECIFIC FIRE AND OTHER SITE PROTECTION INFORMATION			
Type of System or Service Used	**Areas in Operation**	**How Activated**	**Control Panel Location**
Smoke / Heat Detection			
Emergency Alarm for Employee Notifications			
Automatic Fire Alarm Warning System			
Computer or Electronic Room Fire Protection			
Sprinkler System			
Fire Extinguisher Service			
Entry Alarm and Motion Detector Service			
Video Surveillance			
Security / Guard Service			

SERVICE PROVIDER INFORMATION FOR SYSTEM OR SERVICE			
Service Provider Information for System or Service	**Service Provider**	**Phone Contact Day/Night**	**Inspection Cycle Who Performs?**
Smoke / Heat Detection			
Emergency Alarm for Employee Notifications			
Automatic Fire Alarm Warning System			
Computer or Electronic Room Fire Protection			
Sprinkler System			
Fire Extinguisher Service Type of Extinguishers			
Entry Alarm and Motion Detector Service			
Video Surveillance			
Security / Guard Service			

Fire Fighting System Hazards	**Extinguishing Agent Type**	**Health Hazards**	**Needed Employee Protective Actions**
Computer or Electronic Room Fire Protection			
Sprinkler System Extinguishing Agent			
Fire Extinguisher Service Type of Extinguishers and Agents			

Use of Fire Extinguishers

Only use an extinguisher if you have been trained to do so or to escape when trapped by fire. Always note the type of fire the extinguisher is made for before using it on a fire. Basically, fires are classified into the following four types:

- Class A fires occur in ordinary materials, such as wood, paper, excelsior, rags, and rubbish.

- Class B fires occur in the vapor-air mixture over the surface of flammable liquids, such as gasoline, oil, grease, paints, and thinners.

- Class C fires occur in or near energized electrical equipment where non-conducting extinguishing agents must be used.

- Class D fires occur in combustible metals such as magnesium, titanium, zirconium, lithium, potassium, and sodium.

On your floor diagrams note the locations of fire extinguishers, fire-suppression equipment, pull alarms, and exit points. For floor plans at your location contact: _______________________

____

[To the Emergency Planner: Supply contact information for your facility.]

FACILITY SPRINKLER SYSTEM

Manufacturer: ___________________________ Repair number: _______________________

Activated by: ____

Areas located: ____

Other information: ____

CHEMICAL EXTINGUISHING SYSTEM

Manufacturer: ___________________________ Repair number: _______________________

Activated by: ____

Areas located: ____

Other information: ____

Fire Extinguisher Provider: ____

Contact: ____

Service Provider: ____

Refilling: ______________________________ Monthly Checks: ______________________

Establishing Chain of Command and Response Roles

- Selecting employees for emergency response roles.

- During Normal Working Hours / Outside Normal Work Hour

[To the Emergency Planner: This section covers the emergency roles and duties of employees as outlined in this plan. Revise or add the specific information for your facility in the areas where it is requested. Assign the appropriate number of employees to ensure adequate coverage for your facility.]

Establishing Chain of Command – NORMAL WORKING HOURS		
Emergency Role	**Name of Person**	**Title or Position**
Emergency Call-In Center		
Emergency Director		
Assistant Emergency Director		
Emergency Coordinator		
Assistant Emergency Coordinator		
Special Response Teams: Detailed in this section under "Special Response Teams"		
All Employees: Detailed in "Duties of All Employees" in this section		

SEARCHERS AND STAIRWELL MONITORS: Expanded duties in this section		
SEARCHERS	**ASSIGN IN PAIRS / PROVIDE NAMES**	**AREA TO SEARCH**
Searchers		
Searchers		
Searchers		
Searchers		
Searchers		

STAIRWELL MONITORS	ASSIGN BY PROXIMITY TO STAIRS Provide Two Names for Each Stairway	STAIR LOCATION Floor / Compass Direction
Stair Monitors		[2nd fl / NE Corner]
Stair Monitors		
Stair Monitors		
Stair Monitors		
Stair Monitors		
Stair Monitors		

ESTABLISHING CHAIN OF COMMAND – OUTSIDE NORMAL WORKING HOURS		
Emergency Role	**Name of Person**	**Title or Position**
Emergency Call-In Center		
Emergency Director		
Assistant Emergency Director		
Emergency Coordinator		
Assistant Emergency Coordinator		
Special Response Teams: Detailed in this section under "Special Response Teams"		
All Employees: Detailed in "Duties of All Employees" in this section		
SEARCHERS and **STAIRWELL MONITORS:** Expanded duties in this section		
SEARCHERS	**ASSIGN IN PAIRS / PROVIDE NAMES**	**AREA TO SEARCH**
Searchers		
Searchers		
Searchers		
Searchers		
Searchers		
STAIRWELL MONITORS	**ASSIGN BY PROXIMITY TO STAIRS** **Provide Two Names for Each Stairway**	**STAIR LOCATION** **Floor / Compass Direction**
Stair Monitors		[2nd fl / NE Corner]
Stair Monitors		
Stair Monitors		

Emergency Director

This person is selected because he or she is familiar with and/or oversees facility activities during normal operations.

[To the Emergency Planner: Select the name/job title of the person from your facility who will function as the Emergency Director.]

Emergency Director: ____

Duties of the Emergency Director

- Evaluates incoming emergency-related information.
- Determines the response plan of action and activates it.
- Notifies and updates upper management of status of the emergency.
- Acts as the official representative of the facility, communicating with outside fire and rescue agencies.
- Supports and monitors emergency activities, and assigns personnel as needed.
- Provides information to media contacts.
- Assists in determining when the resumption of normal activities can begin.

Assistant Emergency Director

The person selected to be the Assistant Emergency Director also needs to be familiar with the facility activities. The designated Assistant Emergency Director will assume the role of Emergency Director in the event of the Emergency Director's absence.

[To the Emergency Planner: Insert name and title of the person designated as Assistant Emergency Director.]

Assistant Emergency Director: ____

Duties of the Assistant Emergency Director

- Evaluates the site of the emergency and assists emergency efforts of facility personnel.
- Communicates directly with the Emergency Director.
- Assists contractors, visitors, and others as necessary.
- Responds to the emergency as necessary.
- Assists outside rescue and fire agencies.
- Ensures that gates and doors are open for outside rescue and fire agencies.
- Ensures guides are posted for outside rescue and fire agencies.
- Knows locations of shut-off valves for all utility services and electrical and communications panels.
- Assumes the role of the Emergency Director when he or she is not available; assigns a temporary Assistant Emergency Director.

Emergency Coordinator

An Emergency Coordinator and an Assistant Emergency Coordinator should be assigned for each department or unit. Their key duties are to instruct new employees on the facility's emergency response procedures, train Searchers and Stairwell Monitors for their department, and perform a roll call in the event of an actual evacuation. It is recommended each department have its own Emergency Coordinator. It is likely the Emergency Coordinator will perform the duties during an event when outside responders are summoned if the Emergency Director is not available.

Emergency Coordinator: ____

[To the Emergency Planner: Insert the names and job titles of people who will assume these duties at your facility. Depending on the size of your operation, the Emergency Coordinator may take on some of the duties of the Emergency Director; for example, meeting with the Incident Site Commander during an on-site emergency.]

Duties of the Emergency Coordinator

- Each Emergency Coordinator must be familiar with all Emergency Response Procedures and may take on the Emergency Director's duties during evacuations to meet with outside responders.

- The Emergency Coordinator will maintain a current list of site personnel for emergency roll call purposes.

- The protection of personnel is priority one. If there is ample time, employees will secure any records of value and confidentiality.

- Based on hours of operation, location, and department size, the Emergency Coordinator will appoint and train the appropriate number of Stairwell Monitors, Searchers, and their alternates. The Emergency Coordinator will maintain a current list of these personnel and appoint replacements as necessary.

- The Emergency Coordinator will ensure that all Special Response Team members have received appropriate training prior to being assigned any special response duties.

- The Emergency Coordinator is responsible for training new department personnel in emergency response procedures as well as annual refresher training.

- In an emergency, the Emergency Coordinator is the department decision maker, initiator, and coordinator of the appropriate Action Plan for the department staff from the location's command center.

- In the event of an evacuation, the Emergency Coordinator will perform a roll call and account for all staff and visitors. The Emergency Coordinator will forward the results of the roll call immediately to the Emergency Director or, if not available, to the responding outside agencies.

Assistant Emergency Coordinator

Assistant Emergency Coordinator: ____

[To the Emergency Planner: Insert names and normal job titles during the regular workday of persons who will assume these duties at your facility.]

Duties of an Assistant Emergency Coordinator

- Performs duties of Emergency Coordinator when the Emergency Coordinator is not available.

- Assists the Emergency Coordinator during emergencies.

Stairwell Monitors

The roles of Stairwell Monitors are vital to an effective facility Emergency Response Plan. Any employee may have to fulfill the function of a Stairwell Monitor. As such, all employees should be trained on these duties because any employee may be the closest person to the stairway during an evacuation and be required to know how to safely open the door.

There will be two Stairwell Monitors assigned to each stairwell entrance equipped with a fire door. Stairwell Monitors will be the trained employees who happen to be closest to the entrance of the fire door when an alarm sounds.

The first monitor who arrives assumes the first five duties listed. Each Stairwell Monitor will be stationed at the stairwell entrance. Stairwell Monitors report to Emergency Coordinators of their departments or units.

Duties of Stairwell Monitors

- During an evacuation, the Stairwell Monitor immediately goes to the nearest assigned stairway emergency exit. Using the back of the hand to check the door for heat, the Stairwell Monitor stands off to the side, carefully opening the door to determine if the stairwell is clear of smoke and is passable. If so, the Stairwell Monitor directs people to use the stairwell in evacuating to the exit at ground level.

- If stairwell is smoke-filled or not passable, the Stairwell Monitor will stay to direct people to alternate exit(s). Monitors will notify their command center as to the status of the stairwell, if it is impassable.

- The monitors will keep traffic moving on the stairs in an orderly manner and keep the talking to a minimum.

- When it is necessary for the fire department to use a designated stairwell, the Stairwell Monitor will redirect personnel to the alternate exit(s).

- The monitors will stay in place until all Searchers have passed and/or use of the exit is completed.

- The Stairwell Monitor will implement the clearing procedure for buildings with multiple floors and a lower level. The number of landings a stairwell has will determine modification of the clearing procedure.

The following is the clearing procedure for building with two or more floors:

- The top floor Stairwell Monitor will join the next floor's Stairwell Monitor when the use of the top floor landing exit is completed. (Basement Monitor will move up to the ground floor).

- These floor monitors will proceed to the next floor down when the use of that exit is completed. This procedure will be repeated until the ground floor is reached.

- Stairwell Monitors will report directly to their Emergency Coordinator.

Searchers

All departments will designate an appropriate number of trained search teams for all shifts and hours of operation.

It is critical that Searchers operate in pairs. If one of the Searchers is missing, another employee may accompany the Searcher. When assigning Searchers to an area, always be sure the areas they search overlap with those of other Searchers. Assign a man and a woman to each team if possible to facilitate entering restroom areas.

Personnel who perform as Department Searchers should inform the Emergency Coordinator if they will be absent for extended times on vacations or in training, so alternates can be designated. Department Searchers will report to their department/unit Emergency Coordinator during emergencies.

Duties of Department Searchers

- Searchers will perform a sweep of their departments or unit areas.
- Searchers will check all normally unoccupied rooms—storerooms, training areas, meeting rooms, restrooms—and areas adjacent to their departments and areas where alarms may not be heard or where speakers are missing.
- Searchers shall carefully check all closed doors for the presence of heat and smoke before opening by checking the door with the back of the hand to detect heat, and standing off to the side when opening doors.
- Searchers will close all open doors in areas they have searched.
- Searchers will inform personnel they come in contact with to evacuate immediately.
- Searchers will inform Stairwell Monitors that all people have been evacuated from their assigned areas.
- Searchers will exit the building, proceed to their assigned assembly points, and report to the Emergency Coordinator of their departments.

[To Emergency Planner: List all Special Response Teams at your facility, when they are to be activated and how they are to respond. Provide an overview of their duties.]

SPECIAL RESPONSE TEAMS OVERVIEW
1. CPR / First Aid Services Team **When Activated:** For medical emergencies **Response Duties:** Provide medical response while waiting for outside responders
2. Rescue Carry Team **When Activated:** During evacuations **Response Duties:** Provide assistance to disabled employees or injured employees.
It is understood by management and the members of all Special Response Team(s) not to respond if in a situation where they may receive fatal or incapacitating injuries. They are to stand down and wait for professional firefighters or emergency response groups to arrive on the scene.

Depending on the size of the facility and the particular operation, there may be one or several teams trained in the following areas at your site:

- Use of various types of fire extinguishers and/or incipient and advanced stage fire fighting
- First aid, including cardiopulmonary resuscitation (CPR)
- Critical operations and emergency shutdown procedures
- Evacuation procedures
- Chemical spill control procedures
- Use of a self-contained breathing apparatus (SCBA)
- Search and emergency rescue procedures
- Assistance to disabled employees

Availability of outside resources, such as professional firefighters and medical personnel will determine the needs of Special Response Teams. Members of Special Response Teams need to be trained and certified in the emergency actions they will perform. Annual training for employees and special inspections or testing of their equipment may be required. Contact the National Safety Council for assistance in this area: (800) 621-7615 or www.nsc.org.

> IMPORTANT: Team members need to know when not to intervene in an emergency. For example, team members must be able to determine if a fire is too large for them to handle, or whether search and emergency rescue procedures should be delayed until they can be performed safely.

Special Response Teams

In an emergency or disaster, the role of the Special Response Teams is crucial. They are the first line of defense in certain emergencies. Team members must be initially trained and must practice their skills as required and have their special equipment serviced as required.

SPECIAL RESPONSE TEAMS OVERVIEW
1. ADD TEAM NAME **When Activated:** **Response Duties:**
2. ADD TEAM NAME **When Activated:** **Response Duties:**
It is understood by management and by the members of the Special Response Team(s), not to respond if in a situation where they may receive fatal or incapacitating injuries. They should wait for professional firefighters or emergency response groups to arrive on the scene.

Emergency Response Duties for All Employees

[To the Emergency Planner: This part of your plan will make continual references to the Director of Emergency Management, Emergency Coordinator, Searchers, and other titles. Alternate titles may be substituted for your facility. All employees need to know and understand their responses. This information can be used as a training aid and should be posted with a map of your site showing stairs, exits, and the assembly area.]

Duties of All Employees

- Know the Action Plans, how you are to be notified, and your response when a plan is initiated.

- Know how to report emergencies and to whom, internally and externally.

- If notified to evacuate, proceed immediately to your designated assembly area.

- Know the location of the nearest emergency exit in all areas you may enter.

- Do not use elevators during an evacuation.

- When fire is present evacuate, avoid breathing smoke, and crawl to the closest exit.

- Assist disabled employees and visitors who are on site during an emergency.

ACTION PLANS	NOTIFICATION	RESPONSE
General Evacuation Procedure	Alarm and/or Announcement	Evacuate to assembly area. If visitors or contractors are on site, assist them to evacuate to assembly area.
Tornado Emergency Procedure	Announcement (or insert your facility's method)	Proceed to "safe area."
Bomb Threat Procedure	Call (insert #) to report	Document call. Use documentation provided in this procedure.
Medical Emergency Procedures	Call (insert #) to report	If trained, give aid.
Hazardous Materials Emergency	By Notification or Announcement	Outlined in Notification or Announcement.
Earthquake or Sudden Structural Failure	Building becomes unstable and/or has collapsed	Take cover in archways or under heavy desk; when movement settles evacuate.
Disabled Employees	All above methods of notification and others as needed.	Assigned employees will assist as needed.

FIRE REPORTING AND ALARM SYSTEMS		
Reporting of Fire	Call (insert #)	Give location and details.
After Hours	Call (insert after-hours phone #)	Give location and details.
All Clear	(Insert)	Return to normal activities.
Remember not every variable can be covered in a written procedure. Use common sense as required. The primary goal is to protect life.		
Know the primary and alternate escape routes from your department, all areas of the building you may enter, and your assigned assembly area.		
IN ALL EMERGENCIES, if no one answers at the inside emergency phone number, **IMMEDIATELY DIAL 911 or your local emergency response number AND REQUEST HELP.**		

SECTION II-C

ACTION PLANS—SITE-SPECIFIC EMERGENCY RESPONSE PLANS

[To the Emergency Planner: In this section you will develop site-specific Action Plans for your location for man-made and natural emergencies. Read the entire Guide before completing the information requested in this section. Then delete prompts and instructions addressed to the emergency planner.]

Changes in personnel, procedures, building design, and phone extensions that can effect the established Action Plans, or employees responding, should be the responsibility of each site, department manager, or business unit to report changes to the Emergency Planner.

It is important for all employees to be trained and to understand all Action Plans that pertain to their site or operation. During any emergency, variables or circumstances may not occur exactly as described in this Guide. As a rule of thumb, employees need to use common sense based on the information they have at the time of deciding a course of action. The number-one objective is to always protect people.

- General Evacuation Procedures
- Alternate Site Relocation Plan
- Weather-Related Emergencies
- Bomb Threat Procedures
- Medical Emergency Response Procedures
- Death Response and Notification Procedure
- Hazardous Materials Emergencies
- On-Site Spill or Release of Hazardous Materials
- Earthquake/Structural Failure Procedures
- Armed Robbery and Workplace Violence Emergency Response Procedures
- Media-Related Events
- Nuclear Power Plant Radiological Event
- Alternate Site Relocation Plan
- Preparing Your Employees for Home Emergencies

GENERAL EVACUATION PROCEDURES

[To the Emergency Planner: Provide site-specific information for your facility where requested. Insert the correct emergency title, Emergency Director or Emergency Coordinator, based on your operation and availability of the Emergency Director.]

[To the Emergency Planner: Insert the Name / Address / Phone for location.]

Responsibilities of All Facility Personnel

All facility personnel must understand the correct emergency response and general evacuation procedures for their location. During an evacuation, all facility personnel must assist members of the public, visitors, and contractors to exit the facility premises.

Use of Evacuation Procedure

The evacuation procedure can be used for a variety of events. All employees should be familiar with it.

- The alarm signal will be activated by the following: (Insert name as designated by your plan.)

  ____

- The alarm for this location is a _____________________ and sounds like _____________

  ____ .

- Upon notification that an evacuation is in progress, all company personnel and visitors will immediately use the nearest emergency exit and proceed to their designated department assembly location.

- Do not use elevators.

- The department Emergency Coordinator will take a roll call.

- The Emergency Coordinator will report these roll call results to the Director of Emergency Management or his alternate. The Emergency Coordinator shall emphasize the names of the people from his department who may still be in the building.

- Visitors will remain with the staff member(s) they are seeing and their names will be reported to the Emergency Coordinator.

- All personnel will stay assembled by department until further instructions are received from their Emergency Coordinator.

However, it is important to note that in some emergencies, employees must deviate from these instructions. Use common sense. For example, if smoke is present, employees need to begin evacuating even if the alarm has not been sounded.

> Note that not all emergencies are the same. In some cases, employees will have to follow a procedure that is different from the facility evacuation plan. Be certain to train and drill employees in this need to exercise common sense above all in emergency situations.

Summary of Duties for Employees

Following are the duties of employees during an evacuation of the facility:

- Emergency Coordinators will oversee the evacuation of their own departments.

- Stairwell Monitors will check for heat and smoke to ensure the exit is safe and will assist in the movement of people. Every employee must be trained to assume the duties of the Stairwell Monitor.

- Department Searchers will only operate in pairs and will check for personnel who initially failed to hear the alarm. They will check for heat and smoke before opening any door.

- Disabled Employees: Assign at least two employees to assist in the event of an evacuation or any other emergency that may occur.

See Section IV for site-specific bulding map and grounds with exit and assembly information for your facility/department.

[To the Emergency Planner: Add any additional information for your facility to this plan or in Section IV.]

ALTERNATE SITE RELOCATION PLAN

[To the Emergency Planner: Provide the site relocation information for your facility.]

If it is determined that your building cannot be reoccupied, your department's Alternate Site Relocation Plan shall be implemented. Our alternate site location is:

____

____

____

____

____

WEATHER-RELATED EMERGENCIES

NOAA and General Communications

Through its mission to protect life and property, NOAA is a government agency focused on weather and all hazards that may effect the lives of every American. Decisions are made each day based on NOAA weather information from the chances of a rain storm occurring to potentially life-saving information during a flood. The National Weather Service is part of the NOAA outreach service and is the sole official voice of the U.S. government for issuing warnings during life-threatening weather and man-made emergencies. To capitalize on this service, having NOAA weather radios at your site will provide additional and needed information during both natural and man-made emergencies.

A NOAA weather radio with a warning alarm and battery backup is advised. Additional radios may be required depending on the size, employee population, and location of a facility. The NOAA weather radio needs to be positioned in an area that is monitored at all times. In the event of a man-made or natural emergency, a NOAA weather radio will alert you and provide updates for your geographic area.

In addition to a NOAA radio, consider having cell phones available for employees, or have a list of the employees' personal cell phone numbers in the event regular phone service is disrupted during an emergency. An issue in all emergencies is trying to maintain communication. By having several sources of reliable communications, emergencies can be responded to efficiently. Having several types of cell phone chargers on hand should also be considered if your site is isolated and your communications back-up plan is to rely on the cell phones of your employees.

Additional NOAA Resources and Direct Links:

National Weather Service (Overview, Resources, Training Opportunities): www.nws.noaa.gov

National Weather Service National Hurricane Center: www.nhc.noaa.gov

National Weather Service Local River and Flood Forecast Offices: www.weather.gov

National Weather Service Pacific Tsunami Warning Centers: www.prh.noaa.gov/pr/ptwc

National Weather Service River Forecast Centers: www.nws.noaa.gov/rivers_tab.html

National Weather Service West Coast and Alaska Tsunami Warning

Thunderstorms, Tornadoes, Lightning: This 20-page resource guide includes information for schools from NOAA, FEMA, DHS, NWS and ARC: www.weather.gov/os/severeweather/resources/ttl6-10.pdf.

Extreme Heat Emergencies

[To the Emergency Planner: Provide site-specific information for your facility where requested in all weather-related emergency Action Plans.]

Temperatures of 90 F (32.2 C) with high humidity may cause the following life-threatening conditions.

Heat Cramps:

Characterized by painful muscle spasms of the leg and abdomen. Use firm pressure on cramping muscles or massage area gently. Allow the person to sip water. If the person becomes sick, do not give more water.

Heat Exhaustion:

A form of shock that occurs when the body loses too much water and too many electrolytes through very heavy sweating after exposure to heat. Symptoms include heavy sweating, light-headedness, dizziness, weak pulse, and cold clammy skin. Fainting and vomiting may occur. Move the person to a cooler place and treat for shock, raising legs 8-12 inches (20-30 cm). Apply a cool, wet cloth. Sips of water are okay. Seek medical attention if vomiting continues.

Heat Stroke:

This results when a person has been in a hot environment for a long period of time, overwhelming the body's sweating mechanism. It is extremely life-threatening. Body temperature must be lowered quickly. Skin is hot, red, and dry. Pulse is rapid or strong. Unconsciousness is likely. Arrange for rapid transport to a medical facility for further treatment. Quickly remove the person from the heat to a cool place. Remove the person's clothing down to the underwear. Soak the victim with water. Give no fluids.

> Important: Do not leave children or pets inside a locked vehicle during mild to hot days. Temperatures can quickly soar inside vehicles to double the temperature outside the vehicle. Beat the heat, check the back seat!

Extreme Cold Emergencies

[To the Emergency Planner: Provide site-specific information for your facility where requested in all weather-related emergency Action Plans.]

Hypothermia:

Life-threatening condition. A person's body core temperature falls when the body cannot produce heat as fast as it is being lost. Condition is marked with slurred speech, stumbling, and drowsiness. If the person's temperature drops below 95° F (35° C), death may occur. Seek professional medical attention immediately. If medical service is delayed, gently wrap person in a warm blanket and cover the head. Do not warm the legs, arms, or extremities of a hypothermia victim as this may cause sudden cardiac arrest.

Frostbite:

Body tissue freezes, marked by a loss of feeling. Seek medical attention immediately. Re-warming of frostbite seldom needs to take place outside a medical facility. Areas of the body subject to freezing are the nose, earlobes, fingers, and toes.

Lightning, Thunderstorms, and Electrical Contacts

Lightning is produced by thunderstorms. Lightning side strikes may occur for 5 to 15 minutes from the center of the storm activity. The general rule from the National Weather Service is if you can hear thunder, proceed indoors. If you are outside, the following practices can provide some protection from lightning strikes. A resource for lightning and thunderstorm safety may be found at: http://www.weather.gov/os/severeweather/resources/ttl6-10.pdf.

Outdoor Lightning Safety Rules

1. Postpone activities promptly and do not wait for rain. Many people take shelter from the rain, but most people struck by lightning are not in the rain.
2. Go quickly inside a completely enclosed building. If an enclosed building is not available, get inside a hard-topped vehicle.
3. Make yourself the lowest point. Lightning strikes the tallest objects. Squat down on the balls of your feet if you are in an exposed area.
4. Keep an eye on the sky. Look for darkening skies, flashes of lightning, or increasing wind, which may be signs of an approaching thunderstorm.
5. Listen for the sound of thunder. If you can hear thunder, go to a safe shelter immediately.
6. If you see or hear a thunderstorm coming, or your hair stands on end, immediately suspend your outside activities and go inside a sturdy building or car. Sturdy buildings are the safest place to be.
7. If you cannot reach shelter, stay away from trees. If there is no shelter, squat down on the balls of your feet in the open, keeping twice as far away from a tree as it is tall.
8. Avoid metal. Avoid leaning against vehicles. Get off bicycles and motorcycles.
9. Get out of the water.
10. Move away from a group of people. Stay several yards away from other people. Do not share a bleacher bench or huddle in a group.
11. Remove jewelry, coins, or other metallic objects that may attract lightning.
12. Stay away from tall objects that attract lightning, such as trees or antennae.
13. If you are in a hard-top vehicle, stay inside the vehicle.
14. Before lightning strikes, hair on the head stands up. Crouch or squat close to the ground, but minimize your ground contact. Keep your feet together.

First Aid/Follow-up for Lightning/Electrical Contact

After someone has made contact with lightning, be sure it is safe to administer first aid. If so, open the person's airway and check for breathing and signs of circulation (breathing, coughing, movement, pulse). If none is present, begin cardiopulmonary resuscitation (CPR). Contact and exit burns may be present on the victim. Seek professional medical help after any contact involving lightning and high voltages of electricity. The severity of injuries caused by electrical contact is not always initially apparent and the victim may seem fine.

If a witness to electrical contact is available, the witness should accompany the victim to the hospital and be available to answer the physician's questions. If electrical contact was made from another electrical source, survey the scene to make sure the victim is free from electrical contact or shut off the electrical power source before assisting the victim. If the source of electric power is unknown, or if it may be on or off, contact your local electric utility company.

FLOODS

[To the Emergency Planner: Provide site-specific information for your facility where requested in all weather-related emergency Action Plans.]

Hazard Assessment

Contact your local emergency management office, or your local floodplain manager, for the details of previous floods in your area and the effect on your facility's location. If floods are a known hazard, the local emergency management office will also provide information about the community evacuation plan and steps your facility can take to mitigate the effects of a flood.

If your facility is threatened by a flood, consider establishing procedures for protecting the employees, shutting down your facility's operations, and isolating the utilities.

Additional information about protecting your property from flooding can be obtained through FEMA's Mitigation Series at www.fema.gov and at the National Weather Service Web site: www.weather.gov

River and flood forecasts are produced at 13 National Weather Service river forecast centers across the country (see the Web site at www.nws.noaa.gov/rivers_tab.html)

River and flood forecasts may also be obtained from the 122 local NWS weather forecast offices (www.weather.gov).

Advanced Preparation

Advanced preparation is needed to mitigate the effects of floods and to protect your facility. Every facility located in a floodplain will have different needs. As an Emergency Planner, you should consider the following items for your facility in preparation for potential flooding:

1. Review your facility's insurance policy coverage.

2. Establish emergency shutdown procedures, including utility shutoff information.

3. Establish emergency power and communication sources if regular utility service is disrupted.

4. Determine a number of evacuation routes to higher, safe areas outside flooded areas.

5. Determine if sandbagging your site is possible. If so, have materials on site or make advanced arrangements to have them delivered.

6. Initiate procedures to protect critical business and computer information. Critical business information includes important records, lists of suppliers, vendors, machinery information, business transactions, computer information, and employee home and emergency contact information. Duplicate critical business information, as determined for your business needs, and store off-site prior to floods and other events that may destroy them.

7. Surrounding areas and neighborhoods will be affected by floodwaters. This may affect the availability of your employees for the emergency needs of your business operation.

Sources: FEMA Mitigation Series on Floods, NOAA Flood Series, American Red Cross)

Flash Flood Safety Rules

- Avoid driving, walking, or swimming in flood waters.

- Stay away from high water, storm drains, ditches, ravines, or culverts. Moving water only six inches deep can knock you off your feet. Move to higher ground.

- Do not let children play near storm drains.

- If you come upon a flooded roadway never drive through it. Turn around don't drown!

For more information on flood safety, please visit: www.floodsafety.noaa.gov.

Emergency Communications

[Note to Emergency Planner: Consider having cell phones available, or have a list of employees' personal cell phone numbers in the event regular phone service is disrupted due to flooding.]

- Have at your site a NOAA weather radio with a warning alarm and battery backup. This needs to be monitored at all times during potential flooding conditions.

- Establish a communications link with local emergency management authorities.

- Update employee contact information (their home phone number and a phone number where they will evacuate to outside the flood area).

- Distribute to employees primary and secondary facility contact phone numbers to call for reporting instructions after the flood.

Local Government Emergency Management Contact: [________________________________]

Primary Phone Number: [________________________________]

Secondary Phone Number: [________________________________]

This Site's Emergency Cell Phone Number(s): [________________________________]

Local Utility Contact Information

[Emergency Planner: Secure in advance phone numbers of departments and field people who work with the utility companies.]

Water Company: ________________________________

Electric Company: ________________________________

Gas Company: ________________________________

Telephone Company: ________________________________

Sewer Provider: ________________________________

City Street Department: ________________________________

County Street Department: ________________________________

Flood Emergency Shutdown and Evacuation

- Management will determine when to issue the order to follow established shutdown procedures to secure and protect the facility from the effects of a flood.

- Selected essential personnel will remain to complete these procedures as long as they are safely able to do so. Transportation will need to be provided.

- Nonessential personnel will be released to evacuate. Off-duty employees will be contacted not to come to work.

- Tell your employees never to enter floodwaters on foot or in a vehicle. Half of all flood-related deaths occur in vehicles. Vehicles become inoperable when water causes electrical system failure. Occupants may become trapped in the vehicle and drown. All downed power lines are to be avoided.

- If the building is subjected to flood damage, gas, water, and electrical power should be isolated.

- All fuel tanks and bottled gases need to be secured and isolated.

- Selected stay-behind crew will check the following systems: status of portable water pumps to remove floodwater, alternate power sources for generators, battery-powered emergency lighting systems, etc.

Food and Water Contamination

Food and drinking water that comes in contact with floodwater needs to be discarded. Boil all drinking water and eating utensils before use.

Red Cross Shelters and Services

Your employees and their families may need temporary housing. The Director of Emergency Management will stay in contact with facility employees to keep them informed and to determine their needs for temporary shelter. In the event of an emergency, contact the Red Cross to confirm the location of the open shelters in your area.

Other services the Red Cross provides include cleanup kits, mobile feeding, vouchers for food and clothing, critical stress debriefing, temporary shelters, damage estimates for FEMA, emergency structure repair, and incident debriefing.

[Note to Emergency Planner: Add the following]

Local American Red Cross (ARC) Chapter Contact:

Day Number: ____

Night Number: ____

ARC's Director Number: ____

Hurricanes/Typhoons

[To the Emergency Planner: Provide site-specific information for your facility where requested in all weather-related emergency Action Plans.]

Background

Hurricanes are severe tropical storms with sustained winds of 74 mph (119 kph) or greater. Hurricane winds can reach 160 mph (257 kph) and extend inland for hundreds of miles. Hurricanes bring torrential rains and a storm surge of ocean water that crashes into land as the storm approaches. Hurricanes also may spawn tornadoes. The National Weather Service issues hurricane advisories as soon as a hurricane appears to be a threat. The hurricane season lasts from June through November. For additional information, see the National Hurricane Center Web site at www.nhc.noaa.gov

Buildings involved in hurricanes become destroyed or heavily damaged once structures are breached. Once high winds enter a structure, pressure builds until an exit is created. Once the exit is created, the wind velocity increases through the exit opening, destroying the structure from within.

Hazard Assessment and Mitigation

Begin the hazard assessment by contacting the local emergency management office for the details of past hurricanes in your area. The local emergency management office will also provide information about the community evacuation plan and steps your facility can take to mitigate the effects of a hurricane.

Mitigation and Preparation Considerations

Advanced procedures and preparation are needed to mitigate the effects of hurricanes and protect your facility. *The Emergency Management Guide for Business & Industry*, recommends the following steps be taken to prepare and protect from hurricanes.

1. Review insurance policy coverage.

2. Establish emergency shutdown procedures (include utility shutoff information). Establish emergency power sources if regular utility service is disrupted.

3. Determine evacuation routes to follow.

4. Check the building codes for possible renovations to add to your structure

   ○ Have board-up materials, tools, and hardware available to protect your facility from weather-related damage:

   ○ Roof gable ends—Cover gabled ends with ⅝-in (1.6-cm) plywood or other material to prevent wind from catching underneath and creating an updraft to rip the roof off your building.

   ○ Roofs can have hurricane protective straps installed to secure the roof to the walls of the building.

   ○ Large service or receiving doors—Check with door manufacturer for retrofit braces or other ways to protect a door against wind and water.

   ○ Cover windows with temporary or permanent shutters.

   ○ Secure doors and brace from the inside.

5. Initiate procedures to protect critical business and computer information.

The Emergency Management Guide for Business & Industry. FEMA Contract EMW-90-C-3348 updated September 23, 1996 and remains in effect as of April 2011.

Hurricane watch: A hurricane watch means that a hurricane is possible within 24 to 36 hours. Stay tuned for advisories. Tune to local radio and television stations for additional information. Be alert to evacuate as advised.

Hurricane warning: A hurricane warning means that a hurricane is imminent within 24 hours. Take precautions at once. If advised, evacuate immediately.

Purpose

In the event of a hurricane, all personnel will respond as outlined in this procedure to protect personnel and property of this facility.

Emergency Communications

[Note to Emergency Planner: Consider having cell phones available in the event regular phone service is disrupted due to hurricanes.]

- Have at your site a NOAA weather radio with a warning alarm and a battery backup. This needs to be monitored at all times during hurricane-watch or hurricane-warning conditions.

- Establish communications link with local emergency management authorities.

- Update employee contact information in case of evacuation.

- Distribute to employees the primary and secondary facility contact numbers to call after the hurricane for reporting instructions.

- Tropical storm/hurricane forecasts and hurricane safety preparedness information are available from the National Hurricane Center Web site at www.nhc.noaa.gov.

Local Hurricane Emergency Management Contact: ____

Primary Phone: _______________________ Secondary Number: _______________________

This Site's Emergency Cell Phone Number(s): ____

Emergency Shutdown

[Note to Emergency Planner: Include your facility Emergency Shutdown Procedure in Section IV]

- Management will issue the order to follow established shutdown procedures to secure and protect the facility from the effects of a hurricane.

- Selected essential personnel will remain to complete these procedures as long as they are safely able to do so. Nonessential personnel will be released to evacuate.

- Check the following systems: Portable pumps to remove floodwater, alternate power sources such as generators or gasoline-powered pumps, battery-powered emergency lighting, etc.

- Secure and brace windows, doors, and large service doors.

Tornadoes

[To the Emergency Planner: Provide site-specific information for your facility where requested in all weather-related emergency Action Plans.]

[Tornado Emergency Planning: It is advised that several all-hazards NOAA Weather Radios with tone alert or Specific Area Message Encoding (SAME) technology be in use on site. Describe where they are located at your facility, as well as the numbers for radio stations and outside agencies.]

Tornado Watch vs. Tornado Warning

The National Weather Service issues tornado watches and warnings for the nation. Knowing the difference between a watch and a warning can be a lifesaver.

Tornado watch: The conditions are favorable for tornadoes to develop in or near the watch area. Keep apprised of weather conditions and be ready to take shelter if a tornado warning is issued.

Tornado warning: A tornado is imminent or occurring in the warned area. Take shelter immediately.

Local radio stations and law enforcement agencies can also be contacted for weather conditions. Nonemergency numbers for the local fire and police departments are as follows:

Police Department: ____

Fire Department: ____

Additional Site-Specific Information

[To the Emergency Planner: Provide other information for your site in the space provided.]

____

____

____

____

____

____

Purpose

In the event of a tornado, all facility occupants must move to a safe area within the building as outlined in this procedure. Go to an interior room; but never to an inside corner. Flying debris collects in corners when a structure is breached.

Tornado Announcement
[To the Emergency Planner: Determine how employees will be notified—either by announcement, over a paging system, or by another alarm.]

In the event of a tornado, an announcement alarm will be sounded. The following is a sample announcement: "A tornado emergency exists—proceed to your safe area." The Searchers will proceed through their areas, ensuring all employees have heard the announcement.

Duties of Employees
The duties of the Emergency Coordinator, Stairwell Monitors, Searchers, and all employees are basically the same as they are in a general evacuation. However, instead of leaving the building, occupants will go to the closest designated safe areas (areas below ground are preferred).

In the safe area, staff will be instructed by the Director of Emergency Management when to kneel down in a fetal position facing a wall and to cover their heads with their arms, until the all-clear signal is given.

If visual weather updates are needed, observers will be posted around the building to watch for funnel clouds.

Safest Areas
It is vital that all employees know there is no such thing as a safe area in the event of a tornado. However, there are *safer* areas within any building. These are identified as follows.

[To the Emergency Planner: Provide information for your facility.]

Safe areas are (list areas):

____

____

____

____

On-Site Utility Services
Identify location of shutoffs and disconnects.

Water: Shutoff is located: _______________________________________

Electric: Breakers/Disconnects are located: _______________________

Gas: Shutoff is located: _______________________________________
(Tools may be required)

The Director of Emergency Management will assign an adequate number of employees to be responsible for shutting off the facility's utility services, including water, electricity, and natural gas, in the event the building structure and/or services are damaged in the emergency. These employees need to have the proper tools and know the shutoff locations for these utilities. If the structure is damaged, it should not be entered until the Director of Emergency Management has approved re-entry.

Backup Emergency Operations Center

In the event of a tornado, the Backup Operations Center is located in a safe area within the building.

[To the Emergency Planner: Provide the information for your facility.]

The Backup Operations Center is located: ____

The Backup Operations Center's phone is ext.: ____

Tornado Best Safety Practices

Best Safety Practices

- The safest place to be is an underground shelter, basement, or safe room.

- If no underground shelter or safe room is available, a small, windowless interior room or hallway on the lowest level of a sturdy building is the safest alternative.

- Mobile homes are not safe during tornadoes. Abandon mobile homes and go to the nearest sturdy building or shelter immediately.

- If you are caught outdoors, seek shelter in a basement, shelter, or sturdy building. If you cannot quickly walk to a shelter, take shelter in a vehicle.

Vehicle Best Practices

- Immediately get into a vehicle, buckle your seat belt and try to drive to the closest sturdy shelter

- If flying debris occurs while you are driving, pull over and park. Now you have the following options as a last resort:

  o Stay in your vehicle with the seat belt on. Put your head down below the windows, covering with your hands and a blanket if possible.

  o If you can safely get noticeably lower than the level of the roadway, exit your car, and lie in that area, covering your head with your hands.

  o Your choice should be driven by your specific circumstances.

Tsunamis (Tidal waves caused by earthquakes)

[To the Emergency Planner: Tsunami (Tidal Wave) Emergency Planning Provide site-specific information for your facility where requested for this Action Plan.]

Hazard Assessment

If your facility is located in a coastal area, you need to contact your local emergency management office for the details of past tsunamis (tidal waves) in your area. The local emergency management office will also provide information about the community evacuation plan and steps your facility can take to mitigate the effects of a tsunami.

Background

A tsunami is a series of waves generated by an undersea disturbance caused by undersea earthquakes, volcanic eruptions, landslides, meteorites, or other events. Starting from the area of the disturbance, the waves will travel outward in all directions. A tsunami may originate from one hundred miles to thousands of miles away. Occurrences are considered to be more common in the Pacific Ocean than in the Atlantic Ocean.

Tsunami Details

- Time between the wave crests can range from 5 to 90 minutes.
- Wave speed in the open ocean will average 450 miles per hour (724 kph).
- Areas of greatest risk are 50 ft (15 m) or less above sea level areas within 1 mile (1.6 km) of the shoreline.
- Tsunamis have reached heights of 100 ft (30.4 m).

Warning Signs of an Approaching Tsunami

- Warning signs are an earthquake or ground rumbling.
- Rapid changes in the water near the shore.
- As the waves approach shallow waters, they appear normal and speed decreases.
- When waves start to reach the coastline they grow to a great height.

Tsunami Warning System

The National Weather Service Pacific (www.prh.noaa.gov/pr/ptwc) and the West Coast and Alaska (wcatwc.arh.noaa.gov) tsunami warning centers monitor disturbances that may trigger a tsunami warning for threatened areas. Business and home owners should listen to the NOAA weather radio and local media for tsunami warnings.

Before a Tsunami

Because evacuation orders may be based on certain numerical information, know the following for your area: the height of your street above sea level and the distance from the coast. Turn off gas and electrical services to your facility.

Evacuation Routes

Post several evacuation routes leading to higher ground, in the event one or more routes are blocked.

Establish a Communication Plan

Encourage employees to have an out-of-state number to serve as a family contact point if local service is disrupted.

During a Tsunami

Withdraw to higher ground. Do not go near the beach or low-lying areas (see FEMA Mitigation Series on Tsunamis).

Purpose

In the event of a tsunami, all personnel will respond as outlined in this procedure to protect the personnel and property of this facility.

Emergency Communications

[To Emergency Planner: Consider having cell phones available in the event regular phone service is disrupted due to a tsunami.]

- Have at your site a NOAA all-hazards radio with a warning alarm and a battery backup. This needs to be monitored at all times. Establish a communications link with local emergency management authorities.

- Update employee contact information in case of evacuation.

- Distribute primary and secondary facility contact numbers to employees to call after the tsunami for reporting instructions.

- Tropical storm or hurricane forecasts and hurricane safety preparedness information are available on the National Weather Service's National Hurricane Center Web site at www.nhc.nooa.gov.

Local Emergency Management Contact: [____]

Primary Phone: [____]

Secondary Number: [____]

This Site's Emergency Cell Phone Number(s): [___________________________]

Emergency Evacuation and Shutdown

- Upon official notification of the time when the tsunami will strike the coastal area, management will issue the order to immediately evacuate the facility.

- Known open evacuation routes to higher ground will be conveyed to employees.

- If there is adequate time available, this site will follow the established shutdown procedures to secure and protect the facility from the effects of a tsunami.

- Selected essential personnel will remain to complete these procedures as long as they are safely able to do so. Nonessential personnel are released to evacuate.

- Check the following systems: portable pumps to remove floodwater, alternate power sources such as generators or gasoline powered pumps, battery-powered emergency lighting, etc.

- Secure and brace windows, doors, and large service doors.

- Shut off and secure utility services.

[Note to Emergency Planner: Include additional information if needed for your facility]

____

Additional Information:

____

____

____

____

Note: A *seiche*, or tidal wave on a large inland lake, may have a similar effect of a tsunami.

BOMB THREAT PROCEDURES

[To the Emergency Planner: Provide site-specific information for your facility where requested for this Action Plan.]

All company personnel should know the procedures for handling a bomb threat emergency. The procedures should be readily available and in the hands of all facility employees who, by reason of their assignment, might be expected to receive a phone call, a verbal or physical threat, or suspicious mail or packages. This category includes all telephone operators, mail handling personnel, receptionists, and secretaries to company officers.

> Note the bomb threat checklist for phoned-in threats. Give this checklist to all employees who receive outside calls. Note that the information on letter and parcel bomb recognition is from the U.S. Postal Service and is also used by overseas U.S. embassies.

Receiving a Threat

- If you receive a call, follow and document the call as outlined in the Bomb Threat Checklist for Phoned Threats later in this procedure.

- Record the time and the exact words of the message with particular emphasis on the description and the possible location of the device.

- Be familiar with Letter and Parcel Recognition Points outlined in this procedure.

Reporting a Threat

- Immediately call your Emergency Coordinator. He or she will contact:

[To the Emergency Planner: Add the number(s) for your facility.]

____

- Local law enforcement agency will be contacted immediately by:

[To the Emergency Planner: Add the title/department.]

____

Deciding to Evacuate

Immediately after evaluating the threat, law enforcement agencies will decide whether there might be validity to the threat. If you or they determine the threat is valid, activate your facility Evacuation Procedure.

[To the Emergency Planner: Familiarize staff members who receive incoming calls with the steps to take if a threat is received and how to document it.]

Evaluating and Documenting the Threat

The majority of bomb threats received are crank calls. There is frequently a clue to the validity of the threat in the message itself or in the attitude and manner of the caller. That is why it is important to record the caller's message exactly as it was given. After receiving a threatening call, a Bomb Threat Checklist should be completed immediately after contacting your Emergency Coordinator to report the call.

Deciding if the Threat Is Real

A *bomber*, in placing the call, will usually prolong the call and furnish some detail as to the location of the device and reasons for planting it. The call is frequently repeated.

A *crank caller* tends to be abrupt and hurried. Seldom are details provided regarding the type of device, the location, or the reasons. The crank caller repeats the call less frequently for fear of the call being traced.

What to Do While Speaking to a Caller

Basic instructions are to be calm and courteous. Listen and do not interrupt the caller.

Pretend difficulty with hearing the caller's conversation. Keep the caller talking.

Did the caller appear familiar with the facility or building when he described the location of the bomb(s) or device(s)? If the caller seems agreeable to further conversation, ask questions like the following, documenting his responses.

- What kind of bomb or device is it?
- How many devices did you place?
- When will it/they go off? At a certain hour?
- How much time remains until it goes off?
- Where is it located? In which building? In which area?
- If the building is occupied, inform the caller that if the device detonates (goes off) it could cause injury or death.

Action to Take Immediately After Bomb Threat Call

Notify the: ____ .

[To the Emergency Planner: Insert correct title/department for your facility.]

This person will contact local law enforcement agencies. Company executives will need to be notified.

BOMB THREAT CHECKLIST FOR PHONED THREATS
[To be completed after contacting your Emergency Coordinator.]

Exact message received: ____

____

____

____

____

Name of person receiving call: ____________________ Time: ______ Date: ________

Caller's identity:

Male ______ Female ______ Adult ______ Juvenile ______ Approximate age ______

Origin of call (if you can tell or ask):

Local ______ Long distance ______ Booth ______ Internal ______(from within building)

VOCAL DESCRIPTION			
Accent:	❑ Local ❑ Foreign	❑ Not local ❑ Regional	❑ Other
Language Use / Skills:	❑ Excellent ❑ Fair	❑ Foul ❑ Good	❑ Poor ❑ Other
Speech:	❑ Fast ❑ Distinct ❑ Stutter	❑ Slurred ❑ Slow ❑ Distorted	❑ Nasal ❑ Lisp ❑ Other
Vocal Characteristics:	❑ Loud ❑ High Pitch ❑ Raspy	❑ Intoxicated ❑ Soft ❑ Deep	❑ Pleasant ❑ Other
Background Noises:	❑ Machinery ❑ Bedlam ❑ Music ❑ Voices	❑ Party atmosphere ❑ Trains ❑ Animals	❑ Quiet ❑ Street ❑ Other
Manner:	❑ Calm ❑ Rational ❑ Coherent ❑ Emotional	❑ Righteous ❑ Angry ❑ Irrational ❑ Incoherent	❑ Belligerent ❑ Laughing

Letter and Parcel Bomb Recognition Points

The following are letter and parcel bomb recognition points.

- Foreign mail, air mail, and/or special delivery
- Restrictive markings, such as "confidential" or "personal"
- Excessive postage
- Hand written or poorly typed addresses
- Incorrect titles
- Titles but no names
- Misspellings of common words
- Oily stains or discolorations
- No return address
- Excessive weight
- Rigid envelope
- Lopsided or uneven envelope
- Protruding wires or tinfoil
- Excessive securing material, such as masking tape or string
- Visual distractions

Action to Take after Receiving Suspicious Package or Encountering a Vehicle with Explosives

Do not handle the package. Evacuate the area the package is in.

Notify: _______________________________ Extension: _______________________________

[To the Emergency Planner: Insert correct title/department for your facility.]

The Emergency Director will then notify local law enforcement agencies.

Local Police: _______________________________ FBI: _______________________________

County Police: _______________________________ Local Fire: _______________________________

State Police: _______________________________ ATF: _______________________________

SOURCE: NATIONAL COUNTERTERRORISM CENTER / HTTP://WWW.NCTC.GOV/SITE/INDEX.HTML

Terrorist Bomb Threat Stand-Off

THREAT DESCRIPTION	EXPLOSIVES CAPACITY[1] (TNT EQUIVALENT)	BUILDING EVACUATION DISTANCE[2]	OUTDOOR EVACUATION DISTANCE[3]
PIPE BOMB	5 LBS/ 2.3 KG	70 FT/ 21 M	850 FT/ 259 M
BRIEFCASE/ SUITCASE BOMB	50 LBS/ 23 KG	150 FT/ 46 M	1,850 FT/ 564 M
COMPACT SEDAN	500 LBS/ 227 KG	320 FT/ 98 M	1,500 FT/ 457 M
SEDAN	1,000 LBS/ 454 KG	400 FT/ 122 M	1,750 FT/ 534 M
PASSENGER/ CARGO VAN	4,000 LBS/ 1,814 KG	640 FT/ 195 M	2,750 FT/ 838 M
SMALL MOVING VAN/DELIVERY TRUCK	10,000 LBS/ 4,536 KG	860 FT/ 263 M	3,750 FT/ 1,143 M
MOVING VAN/ WATER TRUCK	30,000 LBS/ 13,608 KG	1,240 FT/ 375 M	6,500 FT/ 1,982 M
SEMI-TRAILER	60,000 LBS/ 27,216 KG	1,570 FT/ 475 M	7,000 FT/ 2,134 M

All personnel must either seek shelter inside a building (with some risk) away from windows and exterior walls, or move beyond the Outdoor Evacuation Distance.

Preferred area (beyond this line) for evacuation of people in buildings and mandatory for people outdoors.

[1] Based on maximum volume or weight of explosive (TNT equivalent) that could reasonably fit in a suitcase vehicle.

[2] Governed by the ability of an unstrengthened building to withstand severe damage or collapse.

[3] Governed by the greater of fragment throw distance or glass breakage/falling glass hazard distance. Note that pipe and briefcase bombs assume cased charges which throw fragments farther than vehicle bombs.

Note: The decision to implement steps in this table will be determined by the Public Incident Site Commander.

Recommendations for Handling Potentially Contaminated Mail

[To the Emergency Planner: Provide site-specific information for your facility where requested for this Action Plan.]

Mail contaminated by organisms, such as anthrax, can cause infection to the skin, gastrointestinal system, or lungs. For this to occur, the organism must be rubbed into abraded skin, swallowed, or inhaled as a fine, aerosolized mist. Please note that the following guidelines emphasize minimum disruption of suspicious packages and their contents. These guidelines are also basic steps for handling suspected contaminated mail.

General Mail Handling

- Gloves shall be available for use by mailroom personnel.

- Be observant for suspicious envelopes or packages.

- Open all mail with a letter opener or method that is least likely to disturb contents. Do not use bare hands; wear gloves.

- Open packages and envelopes with a minimum amount of movement.

- Do not blow into envelopes.

- Do not shake or pour out contents.

- Keep hands away from nose and mouth while opening mail.

- Remove gloves by turning inside out.

- Wash hands after handling mail.

Suspicious Items

- envelopes with powder or powder-like residue

- postmarks that does not match return address

- restrictive endorsements, such as "Personal" or "Confidential"

- excessive postage

- handwritten, block-printed, or poorly typed addresses

- incorrect titles or title without name

- misspellings of common words

- no return address

- addressed to individual no longer with organization

How to Handle a Suspicious Package or Letter

- Stay calm; put gloves on. Do not shake or empty the contents of any suspicious package or letter.

- Keep hands away from mouth, nose, and eyes.

- Isolate the package or letter.

- Gently cover the envelope or package with anything available nearby (e.g., clothing, paper, inverted trash can, etc.) and do not remove cover.

If Unknown Substance Spills from Package or Envelope

If an unknown substance spills from a package or envelope, do not try to clean up the substance. Avoid creating air currents. Do not handle the package or envelope any further. If material spills on floor, avoid stepping near it. Avoid tracking any spilled materials to other locations. Do not remove any potentially contaminated items from the area.

During working hours, call the Emergency Operations Center at ext. ___________.

Contact the Director of Emergency Management, a representative, or the department ECO or designee immediately. During off-hour emergencies, call (insert name and phone number):

____

Notify others in the room, turn off any fans or portable heaters, evacuate the room, and close the door. Turn off the air movers of heating and cooling systems. Ensure no one enters the room until proper authorities arrive.

Then determine if further action is necessary, such as:

- Report the incident to your facilities security department (Ext. ___________) and to appropriate local and federal law enforcement authorities.

- Report the incident to facility management and building engineers to confirm shutdown of the room's ventilation system.

- List all people who were in the room or area when the package or letter was recognized. Give this list to the health and law enforcement officials.

- Disease can be prevented after exposure to anthrax spores and other biological contaminants by early treatment with appropriate antibiotics.

If you are contaminated, minimize your movements in the suspected contaminated area. This will keep contamination of the building to a minimum. Gently remove heavily contaminated clothing as soon as possible, minimizing dispersal. Wash hands with soap and water.

If shower facilities are available, remove your clothing in the shower under a water stream. Place the clothing into a plastic bag or other container that can be sealed. This sealed clothing needs to be given to responders for proper handling.

MEDICAL EMERGENCY RESPONSE PROCEDURES

[To the Emergency Planner: Provide site-specific information for your facility where requested for this Action Plan.]

Purpose

Medical emergencies can occur at any time. The person finding the victim must first call his facility in-house emergency number to report a serious illness or injury. This allows the person to concentrate on giving initial first aid to the victim according to the level of first aid/CPR training he has received. A call to the in-house emergency number, also allows the Emergency Operations Center to contact trained members of the special response team as well as an ambulance for assistance. Plan to give any outside agencies responding unrestricted access to your facility and to the victim.

The following describes the procedure facility personnel should follow in the event of a serious injury, illness, or death. This procedure covers employees, visitors, contractors, and vendors.

[To the Emergency Planner: The National Safety Council can assist in first aid and CPR training and certification.]

The level of training and number of employees trained is determined by the facility Emergency Planner based on the following considerations:

- Number of employees on site at the facility
- Location of the facility
- Locations of the work sites
- Number of work shifts per workday
- Response time for outside professional medical agencies

Medical Emergency Notification

In the event of a serious injury or illness of a person, contact the in-house emergency number for assistance:

____ .

[To the Emergency Planner: Provide your facility emergency numbers.]

The person taking the call will call for outside assistance, such as an ambulance or the police department. When you make contact with the person at your company's Emergency Operation Center:

- Identify yourself.
- Give the location of the victim and his or her identity, if known.
- Describe the victim's condition.
- Tell whether he or she is breathing and alert.
- State whether paramedics/EMTs are needed.
- If contact with the company's Emergency Operation Center is not possible, the person who finds the victim should contact the appropriate outside agency directly.
- Do not hang up until the emergency operator tells you to do so or hangs up first.
- Send someone to the facility entrance to open doors for the outside rescue agency.

Outside Emergency Numbers

[To the Emergency Planner: Provide the contact information requested.]

Police: ____

Fire: ____

Ambulance: ____

DEPARTMENTAL CONTACT NUMBERS: (CONTACT AS TIME PERMITS)

1. Manager: work ____________________________ home ____________________

2. Director: work ____________________________ home ____________________

3. Public relations: work ____________________________ home ____________________

4. Facility/building mgr: work ____________________________ home ____________________

List locations of first-aid kits and first-aid rooms:

____

____

____

____

____

Initial Response First Aid

- First survey the area to see if it is safe to enter.
- Do respond quickly, using accepted standards of care.
- Do not attempt to move anyone who is unconscious, has a broken limb, or an injured back. Keep the person still.

- Administer first aid as trained. Practice universal precautions.
- Do check for breathing/open airway and administer rescue breathing if needed.
- Do administer CPR, if needed (and if you are trained).
- Do try to stop severe bleeding.
- Do treat for shock and make the patient comfortable. Do get all information concerning the victim and the accident or illness if the person is conscious (signs, symptoms, allergies, medication taken, pertinent past illnesses, last oral intake, events leading to pertinent past illnesses, events leading to the illness or injury).
- If contact was made with blood or body fluids follow the company's Bloodborne Pathogens Standard Exposure Control Plan. If exposure occurs, contact the ___________________

____ .

[To the Emergency Coordinator: Add the title and position.]

- Document the exposure event in writing.
- Do have the victim follow up with a visit to his or her physician.

Note that employees must be properly trained and certified for first aid, CPR, and/or rescue. This is especially true for employees who will respond to medical emergencies. The National Safety Council's First Aid Institute can assist in this training and certification process. The level of training and number of employees trained needs to be determined by the facility Emergency Planner based on the following considerations:

- Number of employees on site at the facility
- Location of the facility
- Locations of the work sites
- Number of work shifts per workday
- Response time for outside professional medical agencies

DEATH RESPONSE AND NOTIFICATION PROCEDURE

[To the Emergency Planner: Provide site-specific information for your facility where requested for this Action Plan.]

Upon discovering a person who is dead, contact your immediate supervisor and provide:

1. Location of body.
2. Name of the deceased, department, or employer, if known.
3. If known, circumstances related to the death.

Contact the necessary outside local agencies and internal departments. Secure the area and minimize disturbing the area prior to the arrival of the police. Remain with the deceased until the police arrive. Assist police and outside agencies with their investigation.

HAZARDOUS MATERIALS EMERGENCIES

[To the Emergency Planner: Provide site-specific information for your facility where requested. Insert the correct emergency title (Emergency Director or Emergency Coordinator) based on your operation and availability of the Emergency Director.]

> Hazardous materials emergencies can affect employees at the facility as well as people in the surrounding communities. Please include special information specific to the hazards at your site. Also include information as required by federal, state, and local agencies.

[To the Emergency Planner: The following is an example of how a company deals with a hazardous materials emergency scenario. Modify it as necessary for your facility location(s).]

- If your location is close to heavily traveled highways, railways, and near various industries, it can be exposed to hazardous materials from an unplanned release.

- The Director of Emergency Management will correspond directly with all federal, state, and local governmental agencies. Therefore, the response will be based on recommendations from these governmental agencies.

- Employees, contractors, and visitors—all building occupants—will be notified and given the course of action to be initiated and the routes to use.

Courses of Action

- General evacuation: Announce evacuation routes to employees. Follow your facility's General Evacuation Procedure. All employees and other building occupants will exit to a predetermined point of assembly.

- Staggered evacuations: The location would be evacuated in sections.

- All building occupants would leave to a predetermined point of assembly.

- Designate restricted areas: Contaminated areas of a location would be evacuated. Employees and other building occupants would be advised as to what areas are deemed "safe."

- Isolate building: If authorities order that people be sheltered in place, employees and building occupants would remain in the building. Outside air sources, such as fans and doors, would be shut down.

At the first opportunity, contact the following departments and personnel:

Director: ______________________________ Home: ______________________________

Emergency Planning Committee Members: ______________________________________

Public Relations: ______________________ Home: ______________________________

Manager: ______________________________ Home: ______________________________

[To the Emergency Planner: In the event your location cannot resume normal activity, your facility Alternate Site Relocation Plan will be activated.]

ON-SITE SPILL OR RELEASE OF HAZARDOUS MATERIALS

Spill

In the event your location has a hazardous waste spill involving (add your site information, e.g., PCBs or oil solvents), follow these steps:

- Call to report the spill as soon as possible to: _______________________________

- If you are trained and can do so safely, stop the source of the spill.

- Contain the spill from entering waterways or drains.

[To the Emergency Planner: Add your emergency number above.]

Air Release

In the event there is release of potentially harmful material such as pipe insulation or gases into the air, follow these steps:

- Evacuate employees, contractors, and visitors (all building occupants) from the immediate area affected.

- Contact the _______________________________ for assistance, at _______________

  ____ .

- If you have been trained to do so, try to stop the source of the release.

[To the Emergency Planner: Add your emergency number above.]

List of On-Site Hazardous Materials

Plan ahead. Develop response plans for hazardous releases from materials you may have on site. This is crucial during new construction or remodeling. List your on-site hazardous materials and their locations in the following table. Per the requirements of the OSHA Hazard Communication Standard (29 CFR 1910.1200), a listing of MSDSs (material safety data sheets) will be maintained:

____ .

[To the Emergency Planner: Give the location(s) where your facility's MSDSs are kept, if not in the Hazard Communication Plan.]

Hazardous Material	Manufacturer	Location in the Facility

[To the Emergency Planner: Add more sheets as needed to complete the hazardous materials list for your facility.]

EARTHQUAKE/STRUCTURAL FAILURE PROCEDURES

[To the Emergency Planner: Provide site-specific information for your facility where requested for this Action Plan.]

> The material in this part of the Guide covers emergency procedures in case of an earthquake or other structural failure. If your facility is in an area prone to earthquakes, advanced preparation is needed to mitigate the effects of such quakes. Examples of this planning include securing bookcases, furniture, and computers. All facility data and information should be backed up at an off-site location. Provide additional site-specific information in this procedure as needed.

In the event of an earthquake or structural failure, there will be very little, if any, warning time in which to react. Advise facility employees, contractors, and visitors (all building occupants) to take the following actions:

- If you are inside, protect yourself immediately by going under the nearest table or desk.

- During the tremors, do not attempt to exit the building. Most fatalities occur when people fail to take cover.

- When tremors have stopped, evacuate immediately. Damage to the structure is likely.

- Follow your facility's general evacuation plan.

- If the building is not to be reoccupied, follow the facility Alternate Site Relocation Plan.

- Do not enter a damaged building until the Emergency Director gives approval to reenter the structure.

> Important note: At the first opportunity, shut off utility service to the building structure if damage occurred. Services should remain off until the building can be inspected.

[To the Emergency Planner: Provide any additional site-specific information for your facility here.]

____

____

____

____

____

ARMED ROBBERY AND WORKPLACE VIOLENCE EMERGENCY RESPONSE PROCEDURES

[To the Emergency Planner: Provide site-specific information for your facility where requested for this Action Plan.]

The next section covers averting and responding to armed robberies at your facility. A Description of Physical Characteristic Form is provided. The form can also be used to record characteristics of perpetrators of other types of criminal activities.

Preventing Robberies

Instruct employees to take the following daily precautions to prevent break-ins and robberies at your facility.

- Check all security equipment.
- Do not discuss cash levels and security procedures outside of work.
- Be alert for suspicious persons loitering in or near the workplace.
- Be alert for unfamiliar or suspicious vehicles near the workplace.
- Report all suspicious activity to your supervisor.

Robbery in Progress

If employees encounter a robbery taking place, instruct them to follow these procedures.

1. Remain calm and avoid any action that might incite the robber to act violently. The robber may be nervous, and further excitement by the employee can cause the robber to panic and harm the employee or bystanders.
2. Obey the robber's instructions, even if it appears that employees cannot be harmed. Money and property are not worth risking a life.
3. Activate a holdup alarm at a safe time, when the robber is leaving. Do not let the robber see the alarm being activated; it may further incite the robber to violence.

After the Robbery

Immediately after the robbery, ensure that no employees have been injured. Once that has been established, follow these steps:

1. Immediately call your local police department.
2. Close and secure the office until the police arrive. This procedure will help preserve the scene of the crime for fingerprints and other physical evidence.
3. Preserve any notes that the robber may have written, such as a request for money or valuables.
4. All employees involved in the incident should write down their own description of the robber and events and should complete the Physical Characteristics Form that is supplied. Employees should not confer with other witnesses or compare notes.

Workplace Violence

[To the Emergency Planner: Provide site-specific information for your facility where requested for this Action Plan.]

Your facility's Workplace Violence Program can be included here. It is important to convey the following information to all employees.

All employees are entitled to a safe and violence-free workplace. If you know of a potential concern or need to report an incident, contact your supervisor or human resources staff at: _______________________________. A copy of this facility's Workplace Violence Policy can be obtained through: ____.

DESCRIPTION OF PHYSICAL CHARACTERISTICS FORM

	Perpetrator 1	**Perpetrator 2**

Male/Female ____

Race/Nationality ____

Height ____

Weight ____

Build ____

Hair Color/Length ____

Glasses ____

Eye Color ____

Scars or Marks ____

Weapon ____
(revolver, automatic rifle, shotgun, etc.)

Jewelry ____

Clothing:
Jacket ____

Shirt ____

Pants ____

Hat ____

Shoes ____

Vehicle:

Type ____

Model/Year ____

Color ____

License Plate ______________________________________

Additional Information on Perpetrator 1: ______________________

Additional Information on Perpetrator 2: ______________________

Do not discuss any details of the event until the police have taken statements from you and your co-workers. Thank you for your cooperation.

MEDIA-RELATED EVENTS

[To the Emergency Planner: Provide site-specific information for your facility where requested for this Action Plan.]

The following material describes how a facility should handle the media during any on-site emergency and any type of event may bring the press to your facility. The public is represented by the press, and the news media have a legitimate right to information that may concern your staff and the community. Remember that through the release of factual information by your designated spokesperson, the spread of false information is prevented.

Duties of a Company Spokesperson

To best serve the interests of the facility, someone needs to be designated as a spokesperson. A backup spokesperson also needs to be appointed. If the spokesperson is off site, consider the amount of time it will take to arrive in a reasonable amount of time to "meet the press" on behalf of your facility.

The designated spokesperson should do the following:

- Gather all available information to determine if it is necessary to set up a press headquarters. A press headquarters office can help keep all press people in one area.

- If the incident or disaster occurred at the company facility, set up the press area away from incident area.

- Remain in contact with the press.

- Provide information that is factual.

- Log and record all information given to the media.

- Avoid speculation on causes of events, amount of damage, and seriousness of injuries.

- Never release names of persons to the press. Let law enforcement agencies do so.

- Always stress the positive.

Notifying Relatives of Injured Employees, Contractors, and/or Visitors

When relatives of people injured in an emergency need to be notified, follow these steps:

1. Use a previously appointed member of upper management to notify the relatives of the injured.
2. Determine what occurred, the number of persons injured, and the extent and seriousness of the injuries.
3. Determine where the injured were taken.
4. Once information is obtained, brief the previously designated member of upper management, and have him go to the injured person's relatives' homes or workplaces to notify them of the occurrence.
5. Always do notifications in person.
6. In the event of a fatality, you may want to consider contacting a local funeral home, the American Red Cross, or a nearby hospital to secure the services of a professional grief counselor.

NUCLEAR POWER PLANT RADIOLOGICAL EVENT

Time, Shielding, and Distance

Increased distance from a radiation source or being inside a masonry building (shielding) limits the effects of radiation. Limiting time of exposure is also key to protection. If you are outside or must go outside, limit your time of exposure. You do not want to contact dust or smoke from a detonation neither on your skin nor through inhalation. Listen for emergency information bulletins if a radiological event occurs. Your choice should be driven by your specific circumstances.

If a nuclear event occurs, organizations within a 10-mile radius of a nuclear station can be notified several ways, including siren notification. If you hear a steady siren blast for 3 to 5 minutes, this signals to tune radios to an Emergency Alert Station (EAS). Notification through the EAS will alert you if any protective action is required. Two basic protective actions to take are sheltering and evacuation.

Sheltering Notification

- Bring all people inside building(s).
- Take a roll call.
- Close all exterior doors and windows.
- Turn off any ventilation leading outdoors.
- If inside a school, move into the school's interior area.
- If advised that dust from an explosion is present, cover the mouth and the nose with a handkerchief, cloth, paper towel, or tissues.
- Wait for further notifications from the Emergency Alert Station.

Evacuation Notification

- Bring all people inside building(s).

- Close all exterior doors and windows.

- Turn off any and all outdoor ventilation systems.

- Take a roll call.

- Inform employees they are on EVACAUATION ALERT.

- Explain evacuation and relocation procedures.

1st Scenario

- If evacuation transport is provided, explain the need to remain sheltered until transportation arrives.

- Identify/confirm transportation staging areas when contacted by outside resources.

- After arriving at the relocation center, take roll call and wait for further instructions.

2nd Scenario

- If evacuation transport is not provided, make sure employees are advised when to use their own vehicles to evacuate.

ALTERNATE SITE RELOCATION PLAN

Insert your Alternate Site Relocation Plan to be used in the event your location cannot be used after an emergency. Be prepared to give details to representatives of the media as to why your facility cannot be occupied and where its operations are being moved.

PREPARING YOUR EMPLOYEES FOR HOME EMERGENCIES

(Additional resources: Ready.Gov, American Red Cross, and state emergency agencies.)

During any event that may cause major disruption or destruction, the needs of your employees and their families must be considered. If families are not prepared for an emergency and must attend to family needs, they may not be able to respond as employees.

Educate your employees on how to be ready for short and long-lasting events. Also provide information for those special events that occur in your general geographic location. For example, some residents may experience volcanic disruptions while others may need to prepare for floods as part of their emergency planning.

Home Emergency Planning Checklist

(Additional information can be provided from your state's emergency office, National Weather Service, and FEMA.)

If you are thinking of preparing your home and family for emergencies, the following are some simple steps you can take to prepare for any event. You should plan to supply all your needs for at least one week. As in occupational emergency response planning, focus on three goals: protecting life, protecting property, resuming normal operations.

Protecting Life

Develop a home emergency response plan:

- Involve all family and household members in planning, including babysitters and other household help.

- Discuss all possible exit routes from each room, the building, and your neighborhood.

- Designate a place to meet after the emergency.

- Put emergency numbers beside each telephone.

- Clear hallways and exits for easy evacuation.

- Locate the main water, electricity, and gas shutoff valves. Know how and when to turn them off. Don't turn off gas unnecessarily. (Your gas company should be the only one to turn your gas back on.)

- Account for everyone's needs, especially those with disabilities, children, seniors, and non-English speakers.

- Practice. Conduct emergency drills. Walk through your plan with household members.

- When clocks change in the spring and fall, change your smoke detector batteries, check and rotate your "main kit" and "go bag" supplies, and review emergency response plan information with your family members.

Assemble two types of emergency kits—a *main kit* and a *go bag*. A main kit should include all supplies you and your household members will need to live for at least one week outside your home:

- water: one gallon of drinking water per person per day

- food: ready-to-eat canned foods and juices; items for seniors, infants, and special needs people; high-energy snack foods; vitamins; manual can opener, food storage coolers with latching lids

- personal items: copy of important documents (see list under "Resuming Normal Operations"), contact lenses and supplies, eye glasses, extra batteries for hearing aids, prescription medications, dental needs

- first-aid kit and manual

- tools and supplies: flashlight, radio, extra batteries, whistle, dust masks, utility knife, duct tape, plastic sheeting, pots, pans, mess kits or disposable utensils, cups, plates, camp stove with one week's supply of fuel, etc.

- sanitation supplies: toilet paper, feminine supplies, plastic bags, unscented household bleach, soap, personal hygiene items, diapers, plastic bucket with tight lid, etc.

- shelter, clothing, and bedding: tent, sturdy shoes, one complete change of clothing per person, lightweight raingear; blankets or sleeping bags; plastic ground cloths, warm coats and sweaters; heavy duty gloves, etc.

- special needs: items for seniors, special needs people, infants, children, pets, etc.

A go bag is for use in the event of an evacuation. It should be easy to carry and have an ID tag. Each member of the family should have his own go bag, containing the following items:

- water, food, and a manual can opener

- flashlight, AM radio, extra batteries

- whistle

- dust masks

- first aid and personal medications

- walking shoes, warm clothing, lightweight raingear

- extra hearing aid, glasses, other personal items

- toilet paper, plastic bags, other personal hygiene supplies

- writing paper, pens, tape

- cash in small denominations

Protecting Property

Learn about your community's resources and train so that you can be a resource for your community.

- Take, and have family members take, CPR and first-aid classes.

- Train to become a ham **radio operator.**

- Set up a neighborhood watch group with your local police department.

- Offer your assistance to your local community emergency response planning committee.

Resuming Normal Operations

The following steps and advance planning will help you resume normal operations after a disaster:

- Designate an out-of-area contact person to inform relatives and friends of your status. Try to choose someone in an area unlikely to be affected by the same emergency that affects you. So that you need make only one call, provide your contact person with the names and contact information of people you would like to keep informed of your situation.

- Duplicate your important documents and keep an extra copy with a friend or family member or in a safety deposit box. Documents you might want to duplicate include:
  - o birth certificates
  - o marriage certificates
  - o death certificates of relatives
  - o driver's licenses
  - o passports

- o social security cards
- o wills
- o property deeds
- o prescriptions for medicines taken regularly
- o auto, health, property, renters', etc. insurance information
- o credit cards
- o financial information (savings, checking, brokerage, retirement, etc. accounts)
- o contact information for relatives and friends
- o insurance claim information: inventory of valuables (written plus photographic or video), receipts for larger items showing year purchased and amount paid

Add to the Off-Site Emergency/Disaster Notification List the names of people to be notified in the event of an off-site emergency or disaster. Also add contact information for your employer.

SECTION III
EXERCISES, TEMPLATES, AND RESOURCES

[To the Emergency Planner: Section III is divided into three parts—A, B, and C. The purpose of this section is to use exercises and actual events to check the Emergency Preparedness Program and Emergency Plans to ensure effectiveness.]

In Section III-A, you will learn to use exercises and actual events to achieve desired results.

- Exercise Performance Objectives (Learning from Actual Incidents)
- Types of Exercises or Drills
- How to Control the Hazards in an Exercise
- Evaluating the Exercise
- Using the Information Learned

In Section III-B, you will be provided an overview of common drills and templates to develop Action Plans for the following:

- Evacuation
- Tornado
- Bomb Threats
- Medical Emergencies
- Hazardous Materials
- Armed Robbery
- Site Security

In Section III-C, you will be provided exercise resources to validate and document exercises for future improvements:

- Exercise Planning and Actual Event Documentation Form
- Post-Exercise or Actual Event Meeting Critique Form
- Power Plant Drill Example

SECTION III–A
SETTING EXERCISE PERFORMANCE OBJECTIVES

An organization can wait for an actual emergency event to determine if the Emergency Plan and the Emergency Program are adequate, or emergency events can be simulated as part of exercises and testing.

- Exercise Performance Objectives (Learning from Actual Incidents)
- Types of Exercises or Drills
- How to Control the Hazards in an Exercise
- Evaluating the Exercise
- Using the Information Learned

EXERCISE PERFORMANCE OBJECTIVES (LEARNING FROM ACTUAL INCIDENTS)

Exercises are used to determine the effectiveness of the emergency program, the people, the policies and implementing procedures, the organization, the equipment, and the agreements—often called mutual aid agreements—and other resources needed to perform work as expected. Exercises, if properly evaluated, can provide corrective action to solve problems identified during the exercise. Testing is applied to determine if a specific plan works as expected. Testing may be evaluated by a pass or fail rating or corrective items to solve problems identified during the testing.

An organization should develop exercise performance objectives for exercises and testing. From the developed objectives, the organization should determine the participants, type of exercise or test, and the scope. The type and number of participants should realistically reflect the actual organization and the number of people responsible for action in the case of an incident.

Participants

Exercise performance objectives should contain a specific statement of the participants in the exercise (in larger exercises, the participants could be teams or functional units), performance that is expected of the participants, conditions under which the expected performance is expected to occur, and the criteria on which the performance is evaluated. Evaluation is based on a combination of observing the actual performance and comparing the observations with the criteria to determine if the expected performance was observed; if not, the "difference" between expected and actual performance is the input for corrective action.

Performance

An exercise performance objective must state *exactly* what performance (behavior) is desired and expected. The paragraph that follows labeled, "Unobservable, Required Performance" discusses certain types of performance that is required but cannot be observed; for example, cognitive recall of information previously learned and stored within the memories of the participants.

Condition

The "condition" is the specific circumstance under which the expected, desired performance will occur. Condition could be based on tools to be used, equipment to be operated, other prior performances, such as emergency notification to personnel expected to take actions as designated in the emergency plan, and so forth.

Criterion

The criterion is the standard that is used for comparison to determine if the observed performance is correct. Each organization should identify the criterion that will be used to compare the observed performance to set measurable standards for the specific performance. If the organization does not have established standards for performance, the standards must be developed by another organization or developed, approved, and promulgated internally by the organization. An example of standards developed by other organizations would be NFPA 472 for response to hazardous materials emergencies.

Unobservable, Required Performance

When training is designed and developed, the instructional content includes knowledge, skills, and abilities (KSA). Another way of viewing content is: what we want people to *know*; what we want them to do (*skills*); and, what *abilities* are needed to perform as expected. This breakdown of content reflects human functions as depends on recalling information and applying it to the present situation and taking appropriate action. All human functions are important in performance to support the mission, including those human functions, such as understanding, knowing, and thinking, all of which are not directly observable.

Exercises and testing may involve assessing the acquisition of knowledge and the demonstration of cognitive skills and functions. If the measurement of cognitive skills and functions is desired during an exercise or testing, indicator behavior performance objectives must be used. The indicator behavior is a predictor that the cognitive skills and functions can be performed competently because direct measurement is not possible. When performances involve mental functions, indicator behaviors must be used to determine if the performance of the mental functions meets expectations based on education and experience background.

Competence

Organizations need personnel that possess the necessary knowledge, skills, and abilities (KSAs) and the competence to correctly perform using those KSAs. Exercises and testing can be used to measure and compare to accepted criteria or competence. Competence suggests that personnel not only possess the desired KSAs but also can correctly demonstrate the ability to apply knowledge and skills to achieve intended results.

Reviewing Exercise Objectives

Developing exercise performance objectives should follow a logical process with characteristics identified by the acronym SMART:[1]

- **Specific**

- **Measurable**

- **Attainable**

- **Realistic**

- **Timely**

---

[1] Department of Homeland Security, *Homeland Security Exercise Evaluation Program (HSEEP)*.

TYPES OF EXERCISES OR DRILLS

SEMINAR

Type Seminar (Introductory, Overview, or Education Sessions).

Aim Provides overview of plan to motivate and familiarize participants with team roles responsibilities, expectations, and procedures. Useful when implementing a new plan or adding new staff or leadership.

Benefits Informal, easy to conduct, and low stress. Success depends on the quality of planning.

Issues Participants must perceive the value of the session.

Timelines 14-day planning cycle, 1 hour duration.

Objectives Specific objectives of what performance is expected of the participants as a result of the seminar.

Safety Normal organizational safety program.

WORKSHOP

Type Workshop (Introductory, Overview, or Education Sessions).

Aim Intended to build a specific product, such as a draft plan or policy.

Benefits Requires specific planning including session performance objectives. The objectives must include a specific statement about the end result of the workshop.

Issues Participants must perceive the value of the session.

Timelines 21-day planning cycle, 3 hours duration.

Objectives Specific objectives that identify the "product(s)" of the workshop.

Safety Normal organizational safety program

TABLETOP EXERCISE

Type Tabletop.

Aim Presents limited simulation of a scenario (presented in narrative format) to evaluate plans, procedures, coordination, and assignment of resources. Addresses one issue at a time and allows breaks for discussion. Familiarizes participants with specific roles.

Benefits Practices team building and problem solving.

Issues Somewhat detailed with a medium stress level.

Timelines 14-day planning cycle, 2 to 4 hours duration, and 30 to 60 minutes debriefing.

Objectives At least three performance objectives stated in terms of audience, performance, conditions, and criteria.

Safety The need for additional medical response resources may be identified during the exercise safety analysis. The assignment of an exercise safety officer is not required.

GAMES

Type Games.

Aim Provides practice in decisions required during a disruptive incident.

Benefits Decisions and actions generate simulated responses and consequences. Involves more participants, simulators, and evaluators such as business continuity staff.

Issues Typically detailed and high stress level. Games often make use of technology during delivery and/or in modeling a response to player actions.

Timelines 30-day planning cycle, 4 to 6 hours duration, and 30 to 60 minutes debriefing.

Objectives At least five performance objectives stated in terms of audience, performance, conditions, and criteria.

Safety The need for additional medical response resources may be identified during the exercise safety analysis. The assignment of an Exercise Safety Officer may not be required.

EXERCISE/DRILL

Type Realistic.

Aim Simulates a scenario as realistically as possible in a controlled environment (involes movement of personnel at the actual site for a short period of time), requiring the actual performance of response functions. Testing communications, preparedness, and availability of resources.

Benefits Decisions and actions occur in real time and generate real responses and consequences. Involves more participants, simulators, and evaluators such as local emergency services and media.

Issues Typically detailed and low or moderate stress level.

Timelines 30-day planning cycle, 15 minutes to 3 hours duration, plus 30 to 60 minutes debriefing.

Objectives Number of exercise performance objectives depends on the number of functions involved. There should be no less than three objectives per function.

Safety Exercise Safety Officer should be assigned and a complete Exercise Safety Analysis performed.

FUNCTIONAL EXERCISE

Type Functional.

Aim Simulates a scenario as realistically as possible in a controlled environment (short of moving personnel, equipment, and resources to an actual site), requiring the actual performance of response functions. Testing communications, preparedness, and availability of resources.

Benefits Decisions and actions occur in real time and generate real responses and consequences. Involves more participants, simulators, and evaluators such as local emergency services and media.

Issues Typically detailed and high stress level.

Timelines 30-day planning cycle, 4 to 6 hours duration plus 30 to 60 minutes debriefing.

Objectives Number of exercise performance objectives depends on the number of functions involved. There should be no less than three objectives per function.

Safety Exercise Safety Officer should be assigned and a complete Exercise Safety Analysis Performed.

FULL-SCALE EXERCISE

Type Full scale.

Aim Deploys personnel, equipment, and resources to a specific location for the real time, real-life simulation of a scenario. Incorporates as many functions as possible to test the entire Emergency Plan.

Benefits Evaluates operational capabilities in an interactive manner; facilitates communication and coordination across the organization and the public–private sector.

Timelines 6 to 8-month planning cycle, 6 to 8 hours duration, plus 60 to 90 minutes debriefing.

Objectives Number of exercise performance objectives depends on the number of functions involved. There should be no less than three objectives per function. Full-scale exercises (FSEs) with more than 100 exercise performance objectives are not uncommon.

Safety Exercise Safety Officer plus a team of safety officers should be assigned. The number depends on the activity and locations involved.

HOW TO CONTROL THE HAZARDS IN AN EXERCISE

If an injury occurs during an exercise, the exercise must stop and will have an undesirable outcome—the injury. At best, part of the team is lost because of the injury. At worst, the team member will have to be replaced. If a team member is replaced, the team is disrupted. Training must be restarted with a new team member, and new teamwork relations must be established. The time spent on the exercise might result in the participants learning the wrong objective: "I am going to get hurt if I do it that way." The decision might be reached in error that the tactics and procedures used when the injury occurred are incorrect just because someone was hurt, not because the "wrong" tactic was chosen. Injuring someone during an exercise is not acceptable.

Controlling the Hazards

A simple approach to hazard control should be used when planning and conducting any exercise. The approach consists of four steps:

Step 1 – Identify the hazard
Step 2 – Eliminate the hazard (engineering control)
Step 3 – Control the hazard (time, distance, and shielding)
Step 4 – Incorporate safety into exercise scenarios

Step 1—Identify the Hazard

After the exercise scenario is written and the potential exercise activities are developed, each separate activity should be examined to identify the hazards. The examination should be conducted for each activity individually and the exercise scenario as a whole.

A team should be used to identify the hazards. The team size may vary with the size and scope of the exercise. Requirements for a hazard control team include:

1. knowledge of the people participating in the exercise
2. knowledge of the characteristics of the location of the exercise
3. skill in exercise planning

To borrow a technique widely used by safety professionals, the Job Safety Analysis (JSA), an Exercise Safety Analysis (ESA), can be used. The technique for analyzing the hazards during the exercise is identical to the JSA. The Exercise Safety Analysis uses a similar form.

EXERCISE SAFETY ANALYSIS			
Type of Exercise		**Planned Date**	
Exercise Event	**Hazard**	**Cause**	**Control**

Step 2—Eliminate the hazard (engineering control)

Eliminate the hazard by eliminating exposure to the hazard during the exercise or by selecting an exercise type that includes more simulation. If it is not feasible to eliminate the hazard, the next approach must be to control the hazard. Consider using an engineering control to eliminate (or control) potential exposure to a hazard. For example, placing a sound barrier to eliminate high noise levels from a high-pressure steam pump is an example of an engineering control.

Step 3—Control the hazard (time, distance, and shielding)

The standard approach to controlling the hazard of exposure to ionizing radiation is *time, distance, and shielding*. The same approach can be used to control the hazards during exercises. Minimize the time exposed to the hazard, maximize the distance from the hazard, and maintain a shield from the hazard. During exercise planning, training should be identified as a pre-exercise control that addresses these.

If further safeguards are needed, and the installation of an engineering control is not feasible, an administration control should be investigated. For example, an *administrative control* is having workers wear hearing protection equipment if the *engineering control* of the sound barrier did not eliminate the high noise level around the high-pressure steam pump.

Step 4—Incorporate safety into exercise scenarios

The objective is to protect all personnel and property from the hazard. An organization should implement an approach to hazard control that employs constant vigilance for the hazard that was not anticipated.

An Exercise Safety Analysis (ESA) should be implemented by the organization for controlling hazards. The ESA becomes part of the Exercise Safety Plan (ESP) and involves the following:

- Exercise Safety Officer(s)

- Exercise Safety Plan

- Exercise Stop-Action Word

- Pre-Exercise Safety Briefing

Exercise Safety Officer. The exercise safety officer (ESO) must have *one, and only one*, responsibility during the exercise: safety of all participants. Participants include all people involved (employees, responders, observers, controllers, and evaluators) and all equipment used in the exercise. If the ESO has any other responsibilities during the exercise, the responsibility for safety of all involved is seriously hampered.

The ESO should be competent in recognizing the hazards involved with the exercise and should be an integral part of the exercise planning process. The ESO should lead the exercise safety analysis during the planning process. Depending on the size and scope of the exercise, an assistant ESO might be assigned.

Exercise Safety Plan. To ensure the safety of all participants, employees, the general public, and the environment, the ESO should develop an exercise safety plan. The completed exercise safety plan must be submitted to the exercise planning committee for review; the exercise director must approve the plan but any modifications should be discussed with the ESO. The exercise safety plan should identify the site-specific hazards of each exercise. The controls that will be used to mitigate each of these specific hazards must be identified in the plan.

Exercise Stop-Action Word. The urgent need to stop an emergency exercise may arise requiring all activity to immediately cease. To ensure all participants know when it is time to stop all exercise-related activities, an exercise stop-action mechanism, such as a word or a phrase, should be defined. If the use of an "exercise stop-action mechanism" is planned, all participants must be informed of the phrase and the immediate action that is to occur when the mechanism is activated. The exercise stop-action mechanism should define the signal and how the exercise activity may resume, when the emergency clears. For example, during Exercise POPEYE (the Department of Energy National Exercise for Transportation of Radioactive Material in October 1999), the exercise stop-action phrase was, "POPEYE is out of the box." To resume exercise activity after the actual emergency situation was cleared, the phrase, "POPEYE is back in the box," was used.

Reminder signs should be designed, produced, and distributed. Laminated signs protect against damage and allow for reuse. It is recommended that organizations adopt one exercise stop-action word and continue to use this word during all exercises and testing. Various other terms may be used but all participants must know the word (or phrase) and the immediate actions required when it is heard. The exercise stop-action word should be covered as part of the pre-exercise safety briefing.

Pre-Exercise Safety Briefing. The pre-exercise safety briefing is an integral, necessary part of the exercise hazard control. If a hazard is identified and cannot be eliminated, the first (and some would say the most important) technique in hazard control is awareness. If participants are not aware of the hazard, it is difficult to control the hazard by maintaining distance from the hazard, minimizing exposure to the hazard, and maintaining a shield from the hazard.

All participants must take part in the pre-exercise briefing. The metaphor of the huddle during a sports event is useful for understanding the purpose and importance of the pre-exercise safety briefing. In a "no-notice" exercise setting, the pre-exercise safety briefing may degrade some of desired realism because employees know an exercise is coming, but the exact start time or the scenario does not have to be revealed in advance. In a no-notice setting, the pre-exercise safety briefing can be in the form of a notice to all participating personnel that an exercise is planned and will be conducted.

EVALUATING THE EXERCISE

Evaluators

The evaluators assigned to the exercise (testing) should be knowledgeable of the expected performance. Evaluators should have prepared observation forms that allow for notes to be taken during the event. The exercise performance objectives should be contained on the printed form. Note: Evaluators should not be assigned safety officer duties or as a controller.

Identifying Evaluators

The development of the exercise performance objectives should identify the competencies needed in evaluators. In a multi-organizational exercise, identification of the required competencies should be determined during exercise planning meetings.

USING THE INFORMATION LEARNED

Evaluation of exercises, testing, and actual events should be performed immediately after the conclusion of the event. Evaluations are based on the performance objectives developed to focus and guide the process. The process of evaluation is a two-step process:

1. Observe/measure the performance during the exercise or test.
2. Compare the observations/measurements to the criteria established as part of a properly written exercise performance objective.

The difference between expected exercise performance objectives and actual observed performance is the needed input that will go into the corrective action process. The corrective action process should be evaluated during all future exercises.

SECTION III-B
OVERVIEW/TEMPLATE FOR ACTION PLAN DRILLS/EXERCISES

This section provides an overview of common drills using several types of drill/exercise formats or styles. Always consider the effects of any drill and the impacts it will have on the "critical parts of your operation" that may result in injury to employees, customers, the site, and equipment as outlined in Section II–A.

Evacuation Drill/Exercise

Use Full-Scale Exercise Considerations – Critical equipment monitoring / operation, customer disruptions, etc.

- Sound evacuation alarm.

- Observe employee response.

- Did Searchers operate in pairs?

- Did employees know their assembly area?

- Was a roll call taken?

- Record start and end times of drills.

Tornado Drill/Exercise

Use Full-Scale Exercise Considerations – Critical equipment monitoring / operation, customer disruptions, etc.

Follow these steps and note the following for a tornado drill:

- Test the communication process of informing personnel. How did they receive the tornado warning? Remember that in some cases, a warning may not be received for tornado emergencies.

- Did Searchers operate in pairs?

- Did everyone get to a safe area?

- Were people assigned the task of shutting off utilities?

- Did people charged with shutting off utilities have the tools needed to perform the shutoff?

Bomb Threat Drill/Exercise

Use Functional Exercise

Prevent loss of control and keep drill localized because others may think it is an actual event. Utilize the "exercise stop-action word."

Follow these steps and note the following for a phoned-in bomb threat drill:

- **Before** receiving the call, let Receptionist/Dispatcher (or other staff person) know this is a drill and identify yourself.

- Place the call.

- Proceed with the drill.

- Observe whether the person taking the call recorded the exact message and used the Bomb Threat Checklist to help identify the caller.

Follow these steps and note the following for a suspicious package bomb threat drill:

- Alert the mailroom or other package handlers that this is a drill.
- Deliver the package.
- Observe actions taken when the package handler finds the "bomb."
- Ask the package handler what the next action would be. Would the package handler evacuate the building? Contact the local police?

Medical Emergency Drill/Exercise

Use Drill—Prevent loss of control and keep drill localized because others may think it is an actual event.

Utilize the "exercise stop-action word."

Follow these steps and note the following for a medical emergency drill:

- This drill/exercise should involve trained and certified employees demonstrating their first aid and CPR skills under emergency-like conditions.
- CPR skills can be practiced on a mannequin.
- Note whether participants called for help from outside agencies.

Hazardous Materials Emergency Drill/Exercise

Use Table Top or Drill—Prevent loss of control and keep drill localized because others may think it is an actual event.

Utilize the "exercise stop-action word."

Follow these steps and note the following for a hazardous materials drill:

- Time and practice shutting down the air (ventilation) system and isolating the building.
- Time the length to get to the designated off-site meeting area.
- Make employees aware of the possibility of hazardous material releases from industry or transportation lines, such as highways and railroads.

Armed Robbery/Suspicious Person Drill/Exercise

Use Drill—Prevent loss of control and keep drill localized because others may think it is an actual event.

Utilize the "exercise stop-action word."

Follow these steps and note the following for an armed robbery emergency drill:

- In a meeting setting make sure all participating employees are pre-notified of the subject matter.
- Question participants on steps to take in sounding the alarm, securing the scene, and notifying the proper contacts in your operation.

Test the participants' ability to recall descriptions of people who come in and out of the room.

Site Security Drill/Exercise

Use Actual Drill—Prevent loss of control or disruption

- Observe how guards and receptionists handle people trying to enter or obtain information about your facility.

SECTION III–C
EXERCISE RESOURCES FOR VALIDATION, DOCUMENTATION, AND IMPROVEMENTS

Evaluating exercises not only provides a strong emergency response, it also lays the groundwork for a successful safety program. Documenting drills also is important for successful compliance with government regulations. As a resource, the following two forms and an actual example will assist in achieving these goals.

- Exercise Planning and Actual Event Documentation Form
- Post-Exercise/Actual Event Meeting Critique Form
- Power Plant Drill Example

[Note to Emergency Planner: This form is used for Exercises and Actual Events. For *Exercises* it can be used for planning objectives, setting scenarios, identifying hazards, critiquing, evaluating, and so on. For *Actual Events* it can be used for documenting and critiquing responses. This form may also be used to implement corrective actions into the Action Plans. Follow the prompts and complete the information for either an Exercise or Actual Event. Also note the use of the Five-Point Emergency Strategy. As part of your emergency plan, this strategy can be used to validate the Action Plans.]

Exercise Planning and Actual Event Documentation Form (1-2 pages)

Name of Facility/Type: ____

Address: ___________________ City: _________________ State: _____ County: __________

Manager: _______________________________ Phone: __________________ Ext.: ________

Check one. Exercise: ______ Actual Event: ______

Date: ______ Start Time: _______ End Time: _______

Employees at site: ______ # Employees involved: ______

List All Exercise Coordinator(s) and staff involved.

Identify Exercise(s): Evacuation _______ Tornado _______ Bomb _______ Medical _________

Hazardous Material Emergency _______ Earthquake _______ Robbery _______ Other _______

For an **Actual Event** attach a list all those assigned to emergency duties during the event.

Provide Description of the **Actual Event:**

____

____

____

____

____

Exercise or **Actual Event:** Attach a list of employees participating/involved, and attach roll call lists, etc.

[To Emergency Planner: The following are examples of exercise planning objectives and hazard identification. Complete as a group with a variety of department staff involved. Add objectives as needed. NOTE: Delete the examples when ready to save the form for future use.]

Planning Exercise Objectives/Hazards Identification

To assist the evaluators, review the Five-Point Emergency Strategy for evaluating an Exercise.

Controller/Safety Officer– Mike B.
Evaluator #1   Supervisor Steve T.   **Evaluator #3**   Stocker Tony J.
Evaluator #2   Dispatcher Warren F.   **Evaluator #4**   Warehouse Planner Jack S.

Objectives	Exercise Objective	Condition	Criteria (Evaluation Opportunities)	Evaluators Assignment	Identify Hazards
1	Evaluate new alarm effectiveness, and response of the Searchers/employees during an evacuation	Evacuation of office areas located on 1st fl. prompted by warehouse fires on 5th and 4th floor	• Alarm Effectiveness • Time to evacuate site • Actions of Searchers • Roll-call effectiveness	1 and 2	Very limited hazards for office staff evacuating
2	Evaluate action taken by our fire fighters response to 1st "fire"/ 2nd "fire"	Initial fire response deployment to 5th fl. and notified 4th floor fire is burning	• Routes taken to event • Time to reach event • PPE brought to site	3 and 4	Slips, sprains, strains, and mental stress

Use the Five-Point Emergency Strategy to critique an <u>Exercise</u> or <u>Actual Event</u> in Section II-B.

1) Initial Notifications / Ongoing Communication Process: Describe the initial employee notification process and its effectiveness. Evaluate the communication process during the entire exercise or actual event.

2) Assessment: Observe participants' transition from normal operations to emergency operations. Evaluate the decision process and procedures that are in place.

3) Command & Coordination: Evaluate the effectiveness of the Emergency Coordinator and others charged with decision making and responsibilities during the exercise or actual event.

4) Protective Action: Evaluate the effectiveness of an Action Plan and all participants in emergency roles.

5) Parallel Action: Evaluate the use and involvement of outside responders and resources during an emergency.

[Note to Emergency Planner: This form is used for Exercises and Actual Events. Examples are included for using the form as a post-exercise or post-actual event evaluation tool. Delete the examples when ready and save the form for future use.]

Post-Exercise/Actual Event Meeting Critique Form (1-2 pages)

Meeting Date: _____________ Time: ____________

Location: ____

Attach Attendee List and include Emergency Titles.

Date of Exercise or Actual Event: _________________

Brief description of above: ____

____

____

____

Objective Number 1	Exercise Objective	Criteria	Observations and Identifying Corrective Actions
Supervisor Steve T. Dispatcher Warren F.	Evaluate new alarm effectiveness and response of the Searchers and employees during an evacuation	1. Alarm effectiveness 2. Time to evacuate site 3. Actions of Searchers 4. Assembly-area roll call effectiveness	1. Alarm heard in 90% of office areas on $1^{st}/2^{nd}$ Floor. 2. It took 2 min. 37 seconds to clear the building; one minute faster than the previous drill. 3. Searchers failed to check several areas for employees 4. Assembly-area roll call effective with sign-in sheets

[Note to Emergency Planner: Delete the examples when ready and save the form for later use.]

Corrective Action: Review designated search areas with appointed Searchers.

Person(s) Responsible for Corrective Action Implementation: Steve T.

Date Implemented: March 11

(Notify Emergency Planner when correction is completed.)

Objective Number 2	Exercise Objective	Criteria	Observations and Identifying Corrective Actions
Stocker <u>Tony J.</u> Warehouse Planner <u>Jack S.</u>	Evaluate action taken by fire fighters response to 1st "fire" / 2nd "fire."	1. Routes taken to event 2. Time to reach event 3. Immediate building withdrawal should occur when 2nd fire is reported on the 4th floor	1. Several fire fighters took elevators to 5th fl. This is a violation of our procedures. 2. Time to respond and reach floor was 5 min. by foot 3. Fire Captain split forces to fight fires on both 4th and 5th floor. This is a violation of procedures.

Corrective Actions Identified:

1. Review use of elevators during fires with all employees.
2. Review with fire fighters the policy to withdraw when multiple-floor fires occur.
3. Review that an escape route must always be maintained.

Person(s) Responsible for Corrective Action Implementation: <u>Tony J.</u> / <u>Jack S.</u>

Date Implemented: April 8

(Notify Emergency Planner when correction is completed.)

Objective # & Evaluators	Exercise Objective	Criteria	Observations and Identifying Corrective Actions

Corrective Actions Identified:

____

____

____

____

____

Person(s) Responsible for Corrective Action Implementation: ______________________

Date Implemented: _______________

(Notify Emergency Planner when correction is completed.)

Coal-Fired Power Station Exercise

The following is an actual exercise that was held in Gary Indiana. Note the use of a modified *Exercise Planning and Actual Event Documentation Form* for planning, setting objectives, identifying hazards, and documenting the exercise. Also used was a modified *Post-Exercise/Actual Event Meeting Critique Form* and the *Five-Point Emergency Strategy* to identify what worked and what did not.

Background: FVGS Generating Station employees and local responders planned an exercise with built-in safeguards to avoid disrupting critical operations.

Goals and Objectives	Exercise Objectives and Conditions	Evaluators/ Assignment	Identify Hazards
1	Evaluate the initial and backup fire responder's actions, response time, etc.	Gary Fire Department	Moderate level of hazards as workers respond
2	Observe first aid response in realistic station conditions.	NWI AMERICAN Red Cross	Hazard level low
3	Test the station's evacuation procedure and accounting of personnel.	FVGS Safety Department	Hazard level low
4	Using the five points of the emergency strategy, critique communications and command coordination	FVGS Security Department	Hazard level low

900 Hundred Hours: Exercise Safety Officer (ESO) reviewed for a final time with drill planners, evaluators, and the local fire department each drill test, time, and area to take place. In the event the drill was to be called off, the exercise stop-action word was "Stand Down—Resume to Normal."

1105 Hundred Hours: Coal Mill Area Event: The on-shift supervisor (OSS) was alerted that a fire had broken out in the coal mill area. The initial fire response alarm and announcement was made requesting initial incipient fire fighters to respond to #4/#5 coal mill area. In less than two (2) minutes, a number of mechanics and operators were on site at the scene of the "fire." It was noted that a number of these initial responders brought fire extinguishers with them to the area. These responders were informed by the Exercise Planners that, as part of the drill, the Relief Supervisor was injured, needed immediate first aid for specific injuries, and needed to be evacuated from the facility. The operators and mechanics quickly located a first-aid kit and stretcher. One individual referred to his *First Aid Pocket Guide* for burn treatment and administered first aid. By 1125 hundred hours, the Relief Supervisor had been treated and successfully transported to the designated outside assembly area.

The Five-Point Emergency Strategy for Additional Objectives (See Section II-B)	
Exercise Objectives Tested • Initial Fire Fighters response • Back-up Fire Responders • Testing of First Aid Skills • Evacuation • Searchers Effectiveness • Roll Call Taking	**RESULTS:** Evaluators FVGS Safety Dept./ARC • 2-minute response to location of Fire • 1 to 3-minute response • Excellent – (Responses evaluated by Red Cross) • Immediate • 10 minutes to search required areas • 4 minutes
Improvement Recommendations/Identified Items for Corrections	
• Have an assigned area marked for each department in the assembly area. • Place a *First Aid Pocket Guide* and several pairs of gloves in each first-aid kit. • Searchers need to work in pairs. More search teams are needed to cover areas faster. • Emphasize meaning of various alarms to employees. FVGS Safety Department and Station Emergency Planners together will implement corrections.	

1110 Hundred Hours: Alarm/announcement was sounded twice, requesting back-up fire fighters to assemble in the machine shop to await further instructions. Immediately, 20 mechanics and electricians assembled. At 1113 hundred hours employees were informed that this was an exercise/drill. They were told that several "injured employees" were at the west end of the shop and needed first-aid treatment. They responded by locating three "injured employees," evaluated the injuries, and treated and transported the "injured" to the assembly area.

1118 Hundred Hours: The evacuation alarm was sounded throughout station. Guard force was notified, and internal gates and turnstiles were opened. At 1132 the Gary Fire Department arrived. All personnel proceeded to outside the assembly area where the operator took roll call and radioed results from each department back to the control room where the Gary FD was informed. At 1126 hundred hours, all department personnel are accounted for. At 1138 hundred hours the exercise/drill concluded. Normal activity resumed.

1155 Hundred Hours: The Post Critique Meeting/Exercise Evaluating is held including Exercise Safety Officers, evaluators, and local fire department. Also, the Red Cross and 10 responding station employees who were drill participants met to discuss performance objectives and to identify corrections.

1330 Hundred Hours: The critique was completed.

Additional Resources

The U.S. Department of Homeland Security has developed an extensive exercise program, known as the Homeland Security Exercise Evaluation Program (HSEEP). Volume III (available online) provides in-depth coverage of corrective action and improvement planning. The evaluation guides are available online at:

https://hseep.dhs.gov/pages/1001_HSEEP7.aspx

https://hseep.dhs.gov/support/VolumeI.pdf

SECTION IV-A
CHAIN OF COMMAND, PLAN ENHANCEMENTS, AND SAFETY BRIEFINGS

- Chain of Commands for Various Organizations
  - Single Site Operation
  - Single Site Operation with Multi-Site Buildings
  - Corporate Office with Multi-Site Operations
  - Not-for-Profits, Camp Grounds, etc.
  - City of Hobart, Indiana (Towns, Cities, Counties, etc.)
- Plan Enhancements and Learning Aids
  - Exit, Stairs, And Assembly Information
  - Sample Map of Evacuation Exits and Stairway Information
  - Sample Map of Evacuation Assembly Areas
  - Emergency Response Exam
- Emergency Response Safety Briefings and Teaching Aids
  - Office Site Safety for Evacuation, Tornadoes, and Security
  - Tornado Safety for Office, Field, and Home
  - Site Emergency Reporting Contacts and Chain of Command
  - Employee Response Procedures

CHAIN OF COMMAND FOR VARIOUS ORGANIZATIONS

[To the Emergency Planner: Before you begin to set up your "Chain of Command" structure requested in Section II, review the following examples for different types of operations from single building sites, not-for-profits, and so forth. In the first example, for a single site, there is need for only one chain of command. In the second example, this single site operation has a "main" building and three additional buildings at the same site. If there are different departments or employees assigned to these locations, you may need to assign an Emergency Coordinator, Searchers, etc., for each building.]

Various Operations-Emergency Roles-Responding Structure

> **Emergency Role Overview for a
> Single Site Operation**

Emergency Director
Emergency Coordinator – For each department
Searchers-Each Department or Area – Designated in pairs
Emergency Operations Center
Where emergencies are reported first at your site
Stairway monitors
Needed for multistory sites

Emergency Role Overview for

Single Site Operation
with Multi-Buildings

MAIN BUILDING

Emergency Director
Emergency Coordinator – For each department
Searchers-Each Department or Area – Designated in pairs
Emergency Operations Center
Where emergencies are reported first at your site
Stairway monitors – Needed for multistory sites

| **Building One** | **Building Two** | **Building Three** |

Each Building Needs Designated Employees In The Following Roles
Emergency Coordinator
Searchers – Each Department or Area – Designated in pairs
Emergency Operations Center
Where emergencies are reported first at your site
Stairway Monitors – Where Needed

[To the Emergency Planner: In the following example, the organization has a number of operations. Each site must have an emergency chain of command in place. If the "division" sites have multiple buildings with employees assigned to each, they should have their own emergency chain of command in place.]

Various Operations – Emergency Roles – Responding Structure

Emergency Role Overview for
Multi-Site Operations
Example

CORPORATE OFFICE

Emergency Director
Emergency Coordinator – For each department
Searchers – Each Department or Area
Designated in pairs
Emergency Operations Center
Where emergencies are reported first at your site
Stairway monitors – Needed for multistory sites

Multi-Operating Sites

EASTERN DIVISION 32 Locations	CENTRAL DIVISION 14 Locations	WESTERN DIVISION 44 Locations

Each Location Needs Designated Employees In The Following Roles
Emergency Coordinator
Searchers – Each Department or Area – Designated in pairs
Emergency Operations Center
Where emergencies are reported first at your site
Stairway Monitors – Where Needed

©2011 National Safety Council

[To the Emergency Planner: In the following two examples, each of these organizations has many departments. It may not be necessary or reasonable to organize your full emergency chain of command for each department.

If these departments are in close to proximity to each other in the same building, one Emergency Coordinator may be assigned to cover a number of departments. Searchers and Stairway Monitors may be assigned from these various departments to conduct their roles.

All departments may meet in the same assembly area during an evacuation. The important point is every employee is "assigned" to an Emergency Coordinator during an emergency.]

Emergency Role Overview for
Not-for-Profits, Churches, Camp Grounds, etc.

National Safety Council
Emergency Director
Emergency Coordinator – For each department/operations
Searchers-Each Department or Area – Designated in pairs
Emergency Operations Center
Stairway monitors – Floors 2nd and 3rd

Program Development	Customer Services	Executive & Finance	Conventions & Research	IT, Mail Room and Printing
Publishing	Facilities Operations		Chapters	Defensive Driving
Communications	Foundation		CPR / First Aid	Library Services

Emergency Role Overview for
Town, City, County, etc., Operations

City of Hobart, Indiana

Emergency Director
Emergency Coordinator – For each department
Searchers – Each Department or Area – Designated in pairs
Emergency Operations Center
Where emergencies are reported first at your site
Stairway monitors – Needed for multistory sites

Finance Dept.	Park Dept.	Utility Services	Public Safety
Street Dept.	Engineering	IT Services	Fleet Services

The above operations are located in separate buildings employees are to be designated into these response roles.

Emergency Coordinator
Searchers – Each Department or Area – Designated in pairs
Emergency Operations Center
Stairway Monitors – Where Needed

©2011 National Safety Council

PLAN ENHANCEMENTS AND LEARNING AIDS

Exit, Stairs, and Assembly Information

[To the Emergency Planner: Complete this site-specific information for your facility. This information and your site maps of the building noting exits, fire extinguishers, stretchers, stairs, first-aid kits, and assembly areas should be on maps of your site, included as part of Section II-C for your completed plan.]

EXIT DOOR INFORMATION

EXIT # DOORS: Describe exit-designated doors:

____

____

____

DOOR # 1: Describe where main exit door is located and direction it is facing.

____

____

____

DOOR # 2: Describe where secondary door is located and direction it is facing.

____

____

____

DOOR # 3: Describe where third exit door is located and direction it is facing.

____

____

____

DOOR # 4: Describe where fourth exit door is located and direction it is facing.

____

____

____

STAIRWAY INFORMATION

STAIRWAY # 1: Describe the closest stairway to door # 1.

____

____

____

STAIRWAY # 2: Describe the closest stairway to door # 2.

____

____

____

STAIRWAY #3: Describe the closest stairway to door # 3.

____

____

____

STAIRWAY # 4: Describe the closest stairway to door # 4.

____

____

____

EVACUATION ASSEMBLY AREAS

All personnel will proceed to their designated Assembly Areas.

[To the Emergency Planner: Describe the locations of your facility site-specific assembly area and alternate assembly areas and include them on a map. See examples provided.]

- All personnel will stay assembled by departments.
- Roll call will be taken by the Emergency Coordinator.
- Roll call results will be reported to the Emergency Director.

SAMPLE MAP OF EVACUATION EXITS AND STAIRWAY INFORMATION DETAILS

[To the Emergency Planner: Replace this map with your facility's map. Insert your location's maps at the end of Section II-C.]

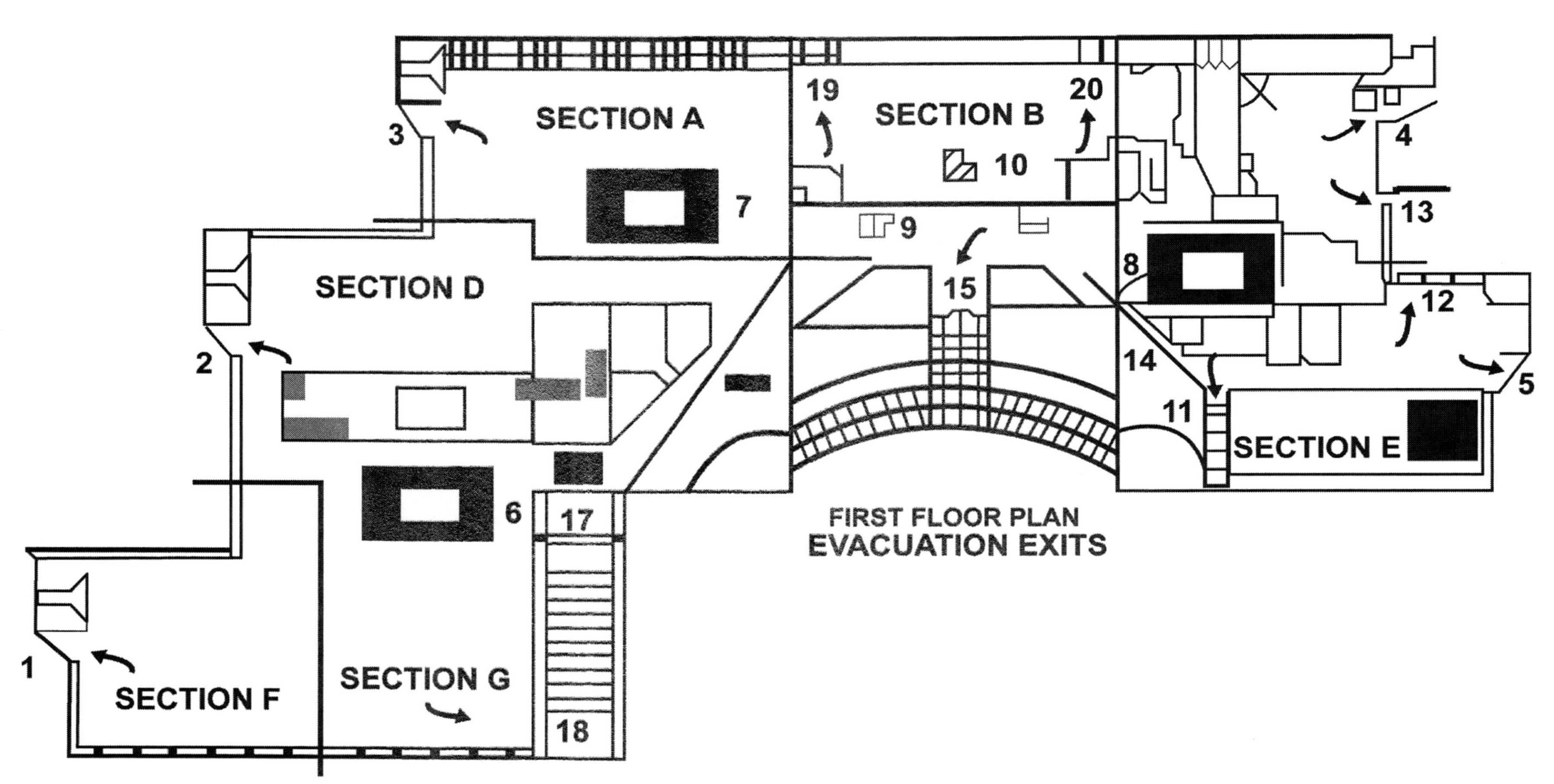

SAMPLE MAP OF EVACUATION ASSEMBLY AREAS

[To the Emergency Planner: Replace this map with your facility's map. Insert your location's maps at the end of Section II-C.]

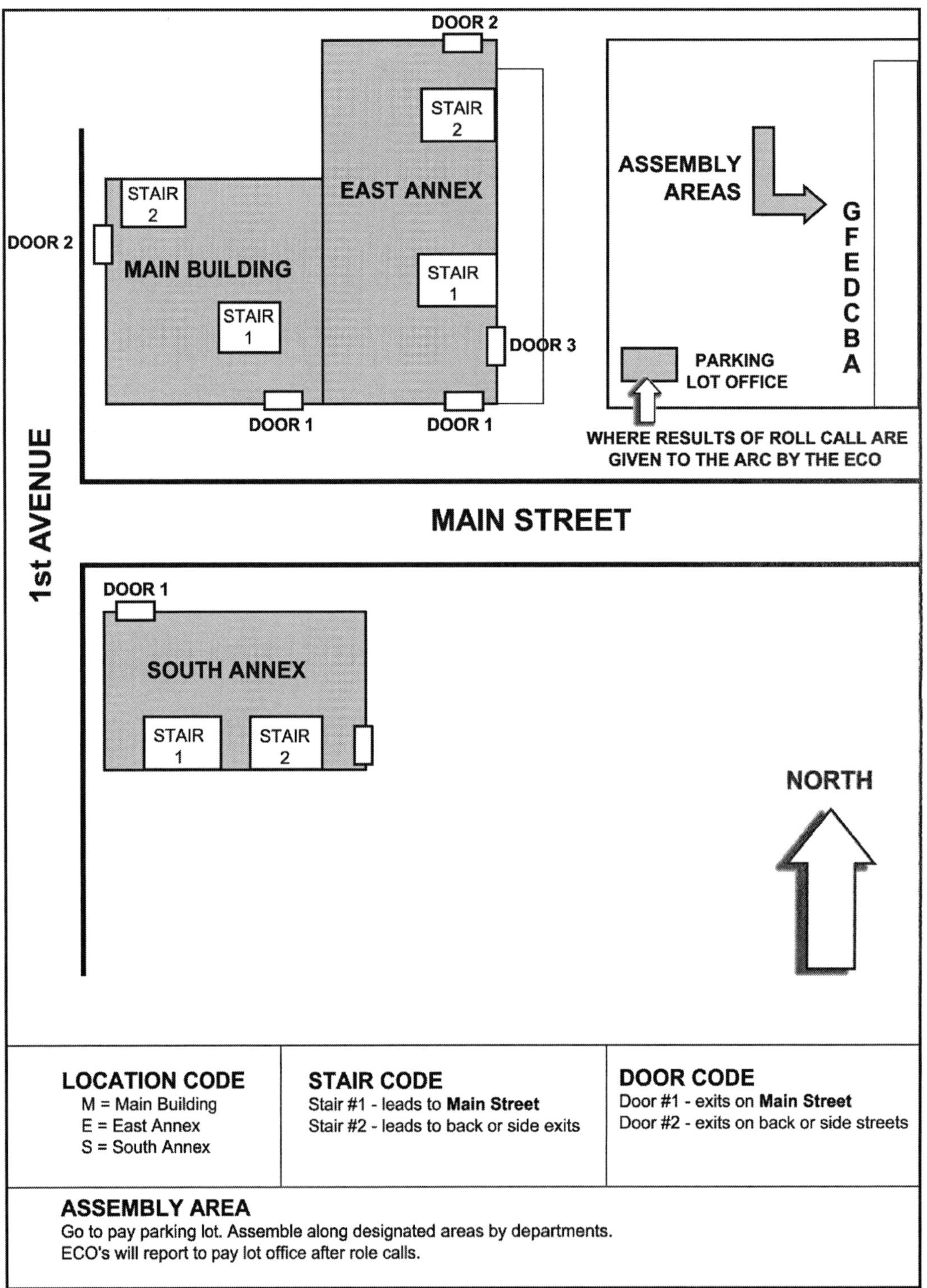

LOCATION CODE	STAIR CODE	DOOR CODE
M = Main Building E = East Annex S = South Annex	Stair #1 - leads to **Main Street** Stair #2 - leads to back or side exits	Door #1 - exits on **Main Street** Door #2 - exits on back or side streets

ASSEMBLY AREA
Go to pay parking lot. Assemble along designated areas by departments.
ECO's will report to pay lot office after role calls.

[To the Emergency Planner: Test your employees before and after training. The goal is to have employees understand what to do and know there is a plan in place.]

EMERGENCY RESPONSE EXAM

1. Who makes the determination to evacuate at your location?

2. What do you hear if a general evacuation of the building alarm is sounded?

3. During an emergency, who is the highest-ranking emergency person at your location? Give this person's title:

4. Your Emergency Coordinator is:

5. What number do you dial to report a bomb threat?

6. Fire breaks out in your work area and it is out of control. After reporting the fire what should your department/business unit do? (Check one.)
   a. Evacuate immediately.
   b. Evacuate only after the evacuation alarm is sounded.

7. Remembering that smoke rises, your work area starts to fill up with smoke. You go to your primary exit and find that it is impassable. The smoke is now waist-high. You should: (Check the one correct answer.)
   a. Hold your breath and run to the alternate exit.
   b. Get under the smoke and crawl to your alternate exit.

8. How are you informed that a tornado emergency exists and you are to go to your safe areas? By:

9. You find yourself next to a stairway exit door on an upper floor when the evacuation alarm sounds. (Check the one correct response.)
   a. You check the door to be sure it is safe to use.
   b. You exit immediately through the door without checking.

10. Safe areas are part of what emergency action plan?

11. Safe areas are located where in your building?

____

12. My department or business unit assembles where outside during an evacuation?

____

13. To report a fire you dial what number?

____

14. To report a medical emergency you dial what numbers?

____

Internally? ____

Externally? ____

15. My alternate work site location is:

____

16. Not every situation can be covered in a written procedure. Employees are encouraged to use common sense. (Circle one.) True or False.

ANSWERS: MOST ANSWERS ARE SITE-SPECIFIC; HOWEVER, ANSWERS TO THE FOLLOWING QUESTIONS ARE LISTED BELOW:

6. A

7. B

9. A

16. True

EMERGENCY RESPONSE SAFETY BRIEFINGS AND TEACHING AIDS

[To the Emergency Planner: Once you develop your emergency response plan it will need to be conveyed to your employees. Your employees must be effectively trained so they understand what actions to take in an emergency. Four safety briefings on emergency responding are included on the companion CD in PowerPoint format. You can revise them for your specific operation's needs. Training can be performed in group meetings, department meetings, and so forth.]

The following slides provide teaching aids on the following topics:

- Emergency office safety for evacuation, tornados, and site security

- Tornado safety for the office, the field, and at home

- Emergency point of contact overview

- Emergency response procedures for employees to know

The Occupational Safety and Health Administration (OSHA) requires documentation of training for employees. Use a sign-in sheet to document a record of those who attend training, or include a place for employees to sign off on the briefings and then collect them. Safety briefings can also be presented as safety posters to ensure employees are reminded of their roles.

Emergency Office Safety for Evacuation, Tornadoes, and Site Security

Emergency and Site Safety for Office Operations
Evacuations / Tornadoes / Site Security

Site Evacuations: Know the following for this site.
1. Evacuation Notification is made by **XXXXXXXXXXXX** for this site.
2. Activate the Emergency Evacuation Plan & Alarm -Searchers operate in pairs.
3. Know the location of the 2 closest exits. Know exits other than your entry door.
4. If you are not located on a 1st floor. Know location of 2 stairways.
5. If a multi-floor site with a landlord. Know landlord's evacuation plan.
6. Know the designated assembly area & title of who is in charge.
    a) If fire is discovered report immediately to those at your site & call 911.
    b) Do not breathe smoke, it can kill. Crawl under smoke to nearest exit.
7. Our assembly area is located: **XXXXXXXXXXXXXXXXXXXXXXXXXX**

Opening Doors During a Fire / Checking a Door for Fire Behind it.
1. Before opening a door, place the back of your hand on the door.
2. Feel for heat and look for smoke around edges.
3. If either are present do not open the door.
Option 1: Call 911. Give your location. Keep smoke out of area with wet towels.
Option 2: If you must evacuate, stand off to the side to open door. Close eyes and hold
    breath. Fire may flash into room.
4. If you need to evacuate, cover head with wet cloth/hold breath. Crawl to exit.
5. Newer multi-level building stairwells may provide temporary safe areas
    for injured or impaired employees to wait for outside rescue.

Tornadoes: Safe areas are located XXXXXXXXXXXXX for this site.

Tornado Watch means tornadoes are possible in your area. Remain alert for
approaching storms. The NOAA Storm Prediction Center issues tornado and
severe thunderstorm watches. **http://www.nws.noaa.gov/**
Tornado Warning means a tornado has been sighted or indicated by weather
radar – time to take cover! Your local National Weather Service office
issues tornado and severe thunderstorm warnings.

Site Entry Security: Display your Identification Badge. Do not let anyone
unknown to you or without the company identification onto site.

If you are approached by people without proper identification, do not let
them in. <u>Contact your Supervisor or On-site Security</u>

For additional information on The Emergency Plan for this
Site, Contact: **XXXXXXXXXXXXXXXXXXX at XXXXXXXXXXX**

©2011 National Safety Council

Tornado Safety for Office, Field, and Home

[To the Emergency Planner: Remember to revise each safety briefing as needed to reflect your specific operation. The information in the following briefing came from the National Weather Service. The information covers work, home, and on-the-road tornado safety.]

Every year the United States has more than 1,000 tornados. They appear suddenly in front of forming thunderstorms. Knowing the correct actions to take, increases your chances for survival. Follow these **National Weather Service** guidelines. It is always important to remember to also use common sense in any emergency.

TORNADO WATCH
➤ Tornadoes are possible in your area
➤ Remain alert for approaching storms

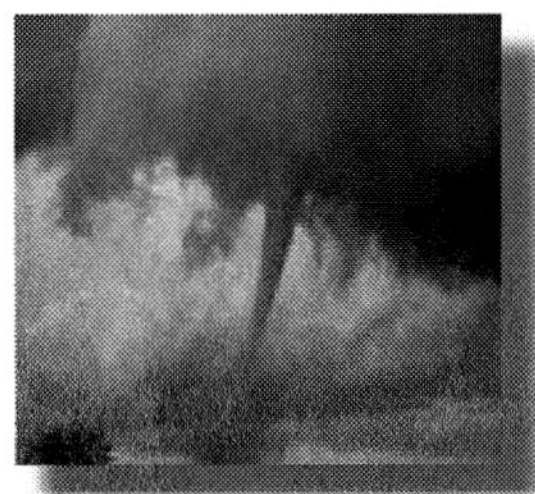

TORNADO WARNING
➤A tornado has been sighted or indicated by weather radar
➤Take cover immediately

Seeking Shelter

Increase survival odds by knowing your shelter options at work, home, and on the road.

WHEN INSIDE – Know the Location of Your Tornado Shelter Areas
1st Choice: Underground shelter (like a basement), then under a table.
2nd Choice: Interior, windowless rooms located on first floor, then under a table.
3rd Choice: Restrooms, closets, hallways with no windows, then close door.
Remember there is no true safe area in a tornado but there are safer ones.

Once in a Protected Area, Take These Extra Safety Steps:
✓ In a kneeling position, face a wall, protect your head with your arms.
✓ Seek shelter in room under a heavy desk or table, protect your head.
✓ After the tornado has passed, evacuate the structure and assemble for a roll call.
✓ If employees are missing, relay information to outside emergency agencies.
✓ All employees are to remain until dismissed by outside authorities.

Your Safest Areas
1)
2)
3)
4)

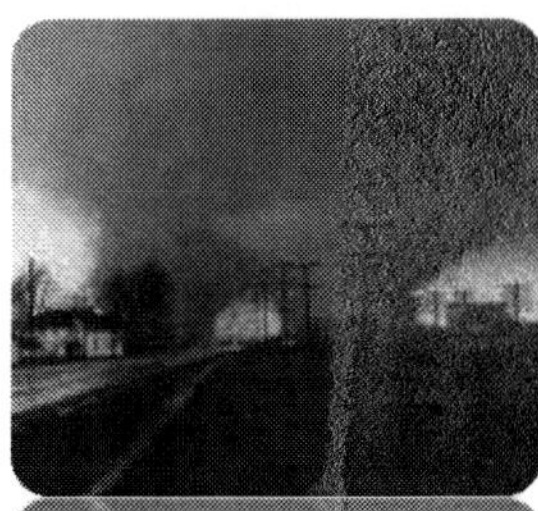

NOAA All Hazards Radios: Homes and businesses need to have these type of radios on-site. The local NWS office issues tornado & severe thunderstorm warnings.
http://www.nws.noaa.gov/

IN A VEHICLE To drive out of the path of a tornado always move at right angles to it.

➤ If you must park, to seek inside shelter, do so as not to block the roadway or traffic lanes.

➤ In some cases, it may be safer to stay in the vehicle. Belt in and stay low. This could be your only choice.

BRIDGES FOR SHELTER
NO WAY! Avoid them. They offer little or no protection against flying debris and are seen as death traps as flying debris ends up in corners.

MOBILE HOMES
➤ Leave the mobile home!

➤ Go to a pre-designated shelter.

➤ As a last resort, lie down in a ditch, depression, or culvert. Lie face down and protect your head with your arms.

IN OPEN COUNTRY
As a last resort, lie face down in a ditch, depression, or culvert. Protect your head with your arms. Stay away from cars, which can roll onto you.

©2011 National Safety Council

Emergency Point of Contact Overview

[To the Emergency Planner: The information below relates directly to what you developed in Section II of this Guide under "Chain of Command" and "Emergency Reporting." This topic also is part of your Five-Point Emergency Strategy in Section II. To make your plan work, all employees need to know how to report emergencies and who is in charge. OSHA will likely require this information if your facility is inspected.]

Emergency Reporting Contacts For This Site

Location:
Address:
Land Line Phone:

Dial <u>9-911</u> To Report Fire, Police or Medical Emergency
• Non Emergency – Fire Dept:
• Non Emergency – Police Dept:
• Non Emergency – Medical:

Local Area Hospitals

•

•

National Poison Control Number – (800) 222-1222

Chain of Contact: Report all emergencies to: **XXXXXXXXXXXX** at this site.
During normal operations this area functions as the: _______________
During off-hour emergencies, call: _____________________________

Emergency Chain of Command

<u>Emergency Director:</u> XXXXXXXXX <u>Located at:</u> XXXXXX

↓

<u>Emergency Coordinator(s):</u> XXXXXXXXX **Located Here**

↓

<u>Searchers</u> (Operate in Pairs / Cover Assigned Areas): **XXXXXXXXXXXXXXXXX**

↓

<u>Stairwell Monitors:</u> XXXXXXXXX
<u>All employees need to know how to check a door</u>
<u>for smoke and heat before opening.</u>

↓

<u>Material Safety Data Sheets are Located at:</u> **XXXXXXXXXXXXX**
(MSDS) Chemical ingredients in a product, precautions when using it, the
effects of exposures and first aid

↓

<u>Human Relations and Corporate Communications:</u> **XXXXXXXXX**

↓

<u>All Employees Know Your Emergency Response Procedures</u>

©2011 National Safety Council

Emergency Response Procedures for Employees to Know

[To the Emergency Planner: OSHA requires you to plan and train your employees on what actions and responses to take for emergencies likely to occur at your workplace. You will have this information after you complete Section II of this Guide. Revise the following safety briefing as needed with your specific information. Remember to document and keep records indicating your employees have been trained. If major changes occur to your emergency plan, employees must be retrained and updated on changes.]

To All Our Employees
Do You Know Your Emergency Response Procedures?

REPORTING AND RESPONDING SUMMARY FOR SITE EMERGENCIES		
Reporting of Fire	Call (insert #) XXXXXXXXXXX Our site's emergency call center is located at: **XXXXXXXXXXX**	During normal operations it functions as: **XXXXXXXXXXX**
After Hours	**Call (Insert after-hours phone # and location if different from above)**	Provide the following if different from above. Police, fire, and medical phone numbers
All Clear Signal	**Insert how employees are notified**	Return to normal activities.

Remember, not every variable can be covered in a written procedure.
Use common sense as required. Everyone's first goal is to protect life.

Know the primary and alternate escape routes from your department, all areas of the building you may enter, and your assigned assembly area.
IN ALL EMERGENCIES report to our inside emergency phone number: **XXXXXXXXX**
IMMEDIATELY DIAL XXXXXXXXX
911 or your local emergency response number AND REQUEST HELP.

ACTION PLANS	NOTIFICATION	RESPONSE
General Evacuation Procedure	Alarm and or Announcement **Evacuate to assembly area**	If visitors/contractors are on-site, assist them to evacuate to assembly area. Site assembly area is located: **XXXXXXXX**
Tornado Emergency Procedure	Verbal or Mechanical Announcement **(Insert your facility's method)**	Proceed to the your designated "Safest Areas," Restrooms, Storage Rooms, etc. Rooms without windows. Protect your head.
Bomb Threat Procedure	**Call (insert #) to report**	Document call. Use documentation form provided in our procedure.
Medical Emergency Procedures	Call **(insert #)** to report. If no answer call for outside help.	Have those trained provide first aid. Designate employees to meet and direct medical responders to victim.
Hazardous Materials Emergency	By Notification from outside agencies.	Follow notification instructions. If sheltering in place, shut down air movers & isolate outside air intakes.
Earthquake or Sudden Structural Failure	Building becomes unstable or has collapsed	Take cover in archways or under heavy desk, when movement settles, evacuate.
Disabled Employees	All above methods of notification	Assigned employees to assist the disabled or injured.
Armed Robbery or Criminal Activity	Contact supervisor or Call 911 as needed	Document event. Use documentation form provided in our procedure.

Do You Have Any Questions?   Contact: XXXXXXXXXXX at XXXXX
©2011 National Safety Council

- List of Hazards NFPA 1600, 2010 Edition from Disaster/Emergency Management Business Continuity

- Planning for Weapons of Mass Destruction OSHA Evacuation Planning Matrix

- Centers for Disease Control-Radiological Emergency Planning (Dirty Bombs and Practical Responses)

- OSHA Checklist for Compliance with 29 CFR 1910.38 and 1910.165 (Employee Alarm Systems)

- OSHA 1910.38 – Elements of an Emergency Action Plan

- OSHA 1910.39 OSHA Fire Prevention Plans

- FEMA The Federal Emergency Management Agency Overview

- FEMA Offices/OSHA Regional Offices

- FEMA Family Emergency Plan Making

- Ready.gov

- Basics of Survival

- FEMA Independent Study Programs (ISP) for Distant Learning

- FEMA Use of Social Media Tools

- FEMA Comprehensive Planning Guide (CPG 101) Required for Planning for Most Public Sector Agencies

- Homeland Security

- Voluntary Private Sector Preparedness Accreditation and Certification Program

- FEMA Tribal Policy

NFPA 1600 LIST OF HAZARDS

The National Fire Protection Association *NFPA 1600 Standard on Disaster/Emergency and Business Continuity Programs* is the result of 20 years of development by professionals from the public and private sectors and has been enhanced through five editions.

NFPA 1600 is globally unique in that it combines disaster and emergency management with business continuity into a management standard that can be directly implemented without modification in any country. It is appropriate in the private, public, and not-for-profit sectors to prevent, prepare for, mitigate for, respond to, and recover from natural, man-made, and techno-logical hazards while continuing to provide critical services throughout the disruptive event.

List of Hazards from NFPA 1600 Disaster/Emergency Management and Business Continuity, 2010 Edition
(1) Naturally occurring hazards that can occur without human influence and have potential direct or indirect impact on the entity (people, property, environment), such as the following:
(a) Geological hazards (not including asteroids, comets, meteors), as follows: i.   Earthquake
ii.   Tsunami
iii.   Volcano
iv.   Landslide, mudslide, subsidence
v.   Glacier, iceberg
(b) Meteorological hazards, as follows: i.   Flood, flash flood, seiche, tidal surge
ii.   Drought
iii.   Fire (forest, range, urban, wildland, urban interface)
iv.   Snow, ice, hail, sleet, avalanche
v.   Windstorm, tropical cyclone, hurricane, tornado, water spout, dust storm or sandstorm
vi.   Extreme temperatures (heat, cold)
vii.   Lightning strikes
viii.   Famine
ix.   Geomagnetic storm
(c) Biological hazards, as follows: i.   Emerging diseases that impact humans or animals (plague, smallpox, anthrax, West Nile virus, foot and mouth disease, severe acute respiratory syndrome (SARS), pandemic disease, bovine spongiform encephalopathy (BSE, or mad cow disease))
ii.   Animal or insect infestation or damage
(2) Human-caused events, such as the following: (a) Accidental hazards, as follows: i.   Hazardous material (explosive, flammable liquid, flammable gas, flammable solid, oxidizer, poison, radiological, corrosive) spill or release
ii.   Explosion/fire

iii.	Transportation accident
iv.	Building/structure collapse
v.	Energy/power/utility failure
vi.	Fuel/resource shortage
vii.	Air/water pollution, contamination
viii.	Water control structure/dam/levee failure
ix.	Financial issues, economic depression, inflation, financial system collapse
x.	Communications systems interruptions
xi.	Misinformation
(b) Intentional hazards, as follows:	
i.	Terrorism (explosive, chemical, biological, radiological, nuclear, cyber)
ii.	Sabotage
iii.	Civil disturbance, public unrest, mass hysteria, riot
iv.	Enemy attack, war
v.	Insurrection
vi.	Strike or labor dispute
vii.	Disinformation
viii.	Criminal activity (vandalism, arson, theft, fraud, embezzlement, data theft)
ix.	Electromagnetic pulse
x.	Physical or information security breach
xi.	Workplace/school/university violence
xii.	Product defect or contamination
xiii.	Harassment
xiv.	Discrimination
(3) Technologically caused events that can be unrelated to natural or human-caused events, such as the following:	
(a) Central computer, mainframe, server, software, or application (internal/external) hazards	
(b) Ancillary support equipment hazards	
(c) Telecommunications hazards	
(d Energy/power/utility hazards	

Source: Reprinted with permission from NFPA 1600, *Disaster/Emergency Management and Business Continuity Programs 2010 Edition*, Copyright ©2010, National Fire Protection Association.

OSHA RESOURCES

Evacuation Planning Matrix

Recent terrorist events in the United States underscore the importance of workplace evacuation planning. Consequently, OSHA developed an Evacuation Planning Matrix (http://www. osha.gov/dep/evacmatrix/index.html) to provide employers with planning considerations and online resources that may help employers reduce their vulnerability to a terrorist act or to the impact of a terrorist release. Terrorist incidents are not emergencies OSHA expects an employer to reasonably anticipate. However, if a terrorist release does occur in or near your workplace, an effective evacuation plan increases the likelihood that your employees will safely reach shelter.

Because terrorism can impact employers and workers, OSHA is committed to strengthening workplace planning and preparedness so employers and workers may better protect themselves and reduce the likelihood that they may be harmed in a terrorist incident. OSHA continues to work with other federal response agencies, including the Federal Emergency Management Agency (FEMA), the Environmental Protection Agency (EPA), the U.S. Soldier Biological and Chemical Command (SBCCOM), the Centers for Disease Control and Prevention (CDC) and, within CDC, the National Institute for Occupational Safety and Health (NIOSH), to provide accurate, current information in this rapidly developing area of occupational safety and health.

Assessing the Risk of a Terrorist Release

Within the Evacuation Planning Matrix, OSHA draws on the Federal Bureau of Investigation (FBI) definition of *terrorism* and defines *terrorist release* as the release of a chemical, biological, radiological or nuclear material (commonly identified as a Weapon of Mass Destruction (WMD)) or of another hazardous substance, performed as a violent act dangerous to human life and intended to further political or social objectives.

To use this evacuation guidance effectively, an employer must first assess the risk of a terrorist release in the workplace. The level of risk is a combination of workplace vulnerabilities, recognized threat, and anticipated consequences of the event. This kind of assessment is not a typical safety and health evaluation. However, guidance on conducting such an assessment is becoming more widely available. For many employers, *Best Practices in Workplace Security*, a homeland security guide developed by the state of South Carolina and available online at http://www. llr.state.sc.us/workplace/fullreport.pdf [PDF], can offer valuable assistance. Its Worksite Risk Assessment List helps employers assess risk based on the following terrorism risk factors:

> *uses, handles, stores or transports hazardous materials; provides essential services, e.g., sewer treatment, electricity, fuels, telephone, etc.; has a high volume of pedestrian traffic; has limited means of egress, such as a high rise complex or underground operations; is considered a high profile site, such as a water dam, military installation, or classified site; or is part of the transportation system, such as shipyard, bus line, trucking, airline.*

If these risk factors apply to your worksite and cannot be eliminated, you may face greater vulnerability to a terrorist release than do other workplaces. To assess the potential threat and consequences of a terrorist release at or near your workplace, consult local law enforcement, the local FBI, and/or the local emergency planning committee (see EPA's LEPC database online at http://www.epa.gov/ceppo/lepclist.htm). You will need information provided by these agencies to complete your overall risk assessment and to determine which of the three risk zones in the discussion that follows best characterizes your workplace.

Chemical facilities can use the U.S. Department of Justice's Chemical Facility Vulnerability Assessment Methodology, online at http://www.ojp.usdoj.gov/nij/pubs-sum/195171.htm, to assess workplace vulnerabilities. Although this document also discusses threat and consequence assessment, you will still need input from local law enforcement, local FBI, and/or local LEPCs to complete your evaluation.

Using OSHA's Evacuation Planning Matrix

The Matrix is *not* a compliance tool for conducting a comprehensive compliance evaluation of an emergency plan developed to comply with the Emergency Action Plan Standard (29 CFR 1910.38) or the Hazardous Waste Operations and Emergency Response Standard (29 CFR 1910.120(q)). Rather, this document covers the general aspects of emergency planning and includes broad questions to help employers *review* their existing plan in light of an indoor or outdoor terrorist release. The document also offers basic planning and preparedness measures for workplaces in each of three risk zones and on-line resources for assistance. After you complete the terrorism risk assessment, review the description of each risk zone to see where your workplace fits best, then examine the planning considerations for that zone.

OSHA offers this guidance to assist employers and workers who are interested in implementing plans and procedures that may reduce the likelihood of a terrorist incident and reduce the effect of a terrorist release, should a terrorist incident occur at a workplace. However, the guidance does not create legal obligations for employers or create rights for third parties. Legal obligations under the OSHAct are created by statute, regulations, and standards.

Note: If you do not have an emergency plan and want to determine whether OSHA requires you to have one, please see Does Your Facility Need an Emergency Action Plan?

OSHA Terrorist Release Risk Categories

OSHA shows the zones in the shape of a pyramid divided into three sections to represent how the nation's workplaces appear to be distributed within the zones. Based on information currently available, the vast majority of American workplaces are at low risk for a terrorist release, that is, they are in the Green Zone, which is the bottom of the pyramid. The questions, recommendations, and online resources in each risk zone build on those in the zone below it. For example, the Yellow Zone, which is just above the Green Zone on the pyramid, includes both the information in the Green Zone and additional information for Yellow Zone workplaces. The Zones are described as follows:

Green Zone: Workplaces that are not likely to be a target for a terrorist release because they are characterized by limited vulnerability, limited threat, *and* limited potential for significant impact (consequence).

Note: If the workplaces near you seem to be in a higher zone, you may wish to review and implement the planning/preparedness considerations in the Yellow Zone.

<u>Yellow Zone:</u> Workplaces that may be targets because they are characterized by high vulnerability, high threat, or a potentially significant impact (consequence), but not more than one of these.

Note: If the workplaces near you seem to be in a higher zone, you may wish to review and implement the planning/preparedness considerations in the Red Zone.

<u>Red Zone:</u> Workplaces that are most likely to be targets because they are characterized by two or more of the following: high vulnerability, high threat, and potentially catastrophic impact (consequence). Such workplaces need to consider sheltering employees in place as well as evacuation, and may consider assigning some terrorist incident response roles to their own employees.

Note: The color-coded risk levels in this Matrix do not equate to the Threat Levels in the Homeland Security Advisory System developed by the Department of Homeland Security. However, employers that place themselves in the Yellow or Red risk levels may consider implementing sequential preparedness measures consistent with those listed in the <u>Homeland Security Presidential Directive – 3</u> for federal agencies.

Limitations of Guidance

Because of the vast number and types of workplaces in the United States, this Matrix provides broad information applicable to most workplaces. If you want to modify your plan to address specific considerations, you can get additional information from the online resources identified. For additional information about workplace emergency planning, see <u>OSHA's Emergency Response</u> Technical Links Web page.

As a nation, our understanding of the risk of terrorist releases and the agents involved continues to evolve. It is likely that OSHA's recommendations for preparedness, training, and equipment also will evolve. OSHA remains committed to helping employers and workers protect themselves from the risk of terrorism in the workplace and is working closely with other federal agencies to provide employers with current information and guidance.

Radiological Emergency Planning

[To the Emergency Planner: Provide additional site-specific information for your facility for this Action Plan. Choices should be driven by specific circumstances if this event occurs. Listen for emergency information updates to decide courses of action.]

If your organization is located in an urban area of a large city, information to survive radiological exposures from dirty bomb attacks have been developed as resources by OSHA and the Centers of Disease Control. Their Web sites have resources that can help to minimize exposure to radiation and increase the chances of survival.

Radiological dispersal devices (RDD), also known as "dirty bombs," consist of radioactive material combined with conventional explosives. They are designed to use explosive force to disperse radioactive material over a large area, such as multiple city blocks. Around the world, there are many sources of radioactive material, which is not secure or accounted for. Rogue nations and/or terrorist groups can obtain these materials for dirty bombs. These explosive weapons may initially kill a few people in an immediate area of the blast, but are used primarily to produce psychological rather than physical harm by inducing panic and terror in the target population.

After a detonation of such a device the concern should be to protect your employees from the exposure of radiation. Basic safety tips to protect your employees from radiation include the following:

- **Time, shielding, and distance:** distance from a radiation source, or being inside a masonry building, limits the effects of radiation.
- Limit time of exposure: If you are outside, or must go outside, limit your time exposure. You want to minimize contact with dust or smoke from a detonation on your skin as well as breathing it in.

The following questions and answers will help employees understand the steps to be taken for protection. Remember these are general responses to be taken. Your choice should be driven by your specific circumstances. Listen for emergency information bulletins if an event occurs. For more information visit the *The Centers for Disease Control and Prevention (CDC) at:* http://www.bt.cdc.gov/radiation/dirtybombs.asp

Frequently Asked Questions (FAQs) About Dirty Bombs

Organizations have expressed concern about dirty bombs and what they should do to protect employees if a dirty bomb incident occurs. Because your health and safety are our highest priorities, the health experts at the Centers for Disease Control and Prevention (CDC) have prepared the following list of frequently asked questions and answers on this topic.

What is a dirty bomb?

A dirty bomb is a mix of explosives, such as dynamite, with radioactive powder or pellets. When the dynamite or other explosives are set off, the blast carries radioactive material into the surrounding area.

A dirty bomb is *not* the same as an atomic bomb

An atomic bomb, like those bombs dropped on Hiroshima and Nagasaki, involves the splitting of atoms and a huge release of energy that produces the atomic mushroom cloud. A dirty bomb works completely differently and *cannot create an atomic blast*. Instead, a dirty bomb uses dynamite or other explosives to scatter radioactive dust, smoke, or other material to cause radioactive contamination.

What are the main dangers of a dirty bomb?

The main danger from a dirty bomb is from the explosion, which can cause serious injuries and property damage. The radioactive materials used in a dirty bomb would probably not create enough radiation exposure to cause immediate serious illness, except to those people who are very close to the blast site. However, the radioactive dust and smoke that spreads farther away could be dangerous to health if it is inhaled. Because people cannot see, smell, feel, or taste radiation, steps should immediately be taken to protect life.

What immediate actions should I take to protect myself?

These simple steps—recommended by doctors and radiation experts—will help protect people. The steps you take depend on where you are located when the incident occurs: outside, inside, or in a vehicle.

If you are outside and close to the incident

- Cover your nose and mouth with a cloth to reduce the risk of breathing in radioactive dust or smoke.

- Don't touch objects thrown off by an explosion—they might be radioactive.

- Quickly go into a building where the walls and windows have not been broken. This area will shield you from radiation that might be outside.

- Once you are inside, take off your outer layer of clothing and seal it in a plastic bag if available. Put the cloth you used to cover your mouth in the bag too. Removing outer clothes may get rid of up to 90% of radioactive dust.

- Put the plastic bag where others will not touch it and keep it until authorities tell you what to do with it.

- Shower or wash with soap and water. Be sure to wash your hair. Washing will remove any remaining dust.

- Tune to the local radio or television news for more instructions.

If you are inside and close to the incident

- If the walls and windows of the building are not broken, stay in the building and do not leave.

- To keep radioactive dust or powder from getting inside, shut all windows, outside doors, and fireplace dampers. Turn off fans and heating and air-conditioning systems that bring in air from the outside. It is not necessary to put duct tape or plastic around doors or windows.

- If the walls and windows of the building are broken, go to an interior room and do not leave. If the building has been heavily damaged, quickly go into a building where the walls and windows have not been broken. If you must go outside, be sure to cover your nose and mouth with a cloth. Once you are inside, take off your outer layer of clothing and seal it in a plastic bag if available. Store the bag where others will not touch it.

- Shower or wash with soap and water, removing any remaining dust. Be sure to wash your hair.

- Tune to local radio or television news for more instructions.

If you are in a car when the incident happens

- Close the windows and turn off the air conditioner, heater, and vents.

- Cover your nose and mouth with a cloth to avoid breathing radioactive dust or smoke.

- If you are close to your home, office, or a public building, go there immediately and go inside quickly.

- If you cannot get to your home or another building safely, pull over to the side of the road and stop in the safest place possible. If it is a hot or sunny day, try to stop under a bridge or in a shady spot.

- Turn off the engine and listen to the radio for instructions.
- Stay in the car until you are told it is safe to get back on the road.

What should I do about my children and family?

- If your children or family are with you, stay together. Take the same actions to protect your whole family.
- If your children or family are in another home or building, they should stay there until you are told it is safe to travel.
- Schools have emergency plans and shelters. If your children are at school, they should stay there until it is safe to travel. Do not go to the school until public officials say it is safe to travel.

How do I protect my pets?

- If you have pets outside, bring them inside if it can be done safely.
- Wash your pets with soap and water to remove any radioactive dust.

Should I take potassium iodide?

- Potassium iodide, also called KI, only protects a person's thyroid gland from exposure to radioactive iodine. KI will not protect a person from other radioactive materials or protect other parts of the body from exposure to radiation.
- Since there is no way to know at the time of the explosion whether radioactive iodine was used in the explosive device, taking KI would probably not be beneficial. Also, KI can be dangerous to some people.

Will food and water supplies be safe?

- Food and water supplies most likely will remain safe. However, any unpackaged food or water that was out in the open and close to the incident may have radioactive dust on it. Therefore, do not consume water or food that was out in the open.
- The food inside of cans and other sealed containers will be safe to eat. Wash the outside of the container before opening it.

Authorities will monitor food and water quality for safety and keep the public informed.

How do I know if I've been exposed to radiation or contaminated by radioactive materials?

- People cannot see, smell, feel, or taste radiation; so you may not know whether you have been exposed. Police or firefighters will quickly check for radiation by using special equipment to determine how much radiation is present and whether it poses any danger in your area.
- Low levels of radiation exposure (like those expected from a dirty bomb situation) do not cause any symptoms. Higher levels of radiation exposure may produce symptoms, such as nausea, vomiting, diarrhea, and swelling and redness of the skin.
- If you develop any of these symptoms, you should contact your doctor, hospital, or other sites recommended by authorities.

Where do I go for more information?

For more information about dirty bombs, radiation, and health contact:

- <u>The Conference of Radiation Control Program Directors (CRCPD)</u> at 502-227-4543
- <u>The Environmental Protection Agency (EPA)</u>
- <u>The Nuclear Regulatory Commission (NRC)</u> at 301-415-8200
- <u>The Federal Emergency Management Agency (FEMA)</u> at 202-646-4600
- <u>The Radiation Emergency Assistance Center/Training Site (REAC/TS)</u> at 865-576-3131
- <u>The U.S. National Response Team (NRT)</u>
- <u>The U.S. Department of Energy (DOE)</u> at 1-800-DIAL-DOE

Links to: <u>OSHA Compliance</u> / <u>Protecting Clean-up Workers</u> / <u>Related Topics</u> / <u>Dirty Bombs</u> / <u>Protecting Surrounding Area Workers</u> / <u>Protecting First Responders</u> / <u>Protecting Health Care Workers</u> RDD Response Organizations / Securing Radioactive Materials / Additional Information /Credits are at: <u>http://www.osha.gov/SLTC/emergencypreparedness/rdd_tech.html</u>

Checklist for Compliance with OSHA 29 CFR 1910.38 and 1910.165

OSHA Checklist for Compliance with 29 CFR 1910.38 and 1910.165		
	Compliance (Yes or No)	**Corrective Action**
(a) Application. An employer must have an emergency action plan whenever an OSHA standard in this part requires one. The requirements in this section apply to each such emergency action plan.		
(b)Written and oral emergency action plans. An emergency action plan must be in writing, kept in the workplace, and available to employees for review. However, an employer with 10 or fewer employees may communicate the plan orally to employees.		
(c)Minimum elements of an emergency action plan. An emergency action plan must include at a minimum: (1) Procedures for reporting a fire or other emergency; (2) Procedures for emergency evacuation, including type of evacuation and exit route assignments; (3) Procedures to be followed by employees who remain to operate critical plant operations before they evacuate; (4) Procedures to account for all employees after evacuation; (5) Procedures to be followed by employees performing rescue or medical duties; and (6) The name or job title of every employee who may be contacted by employees who need more information about the plan or an explanation of their duties under the plan.		

	Compliance (Yes or No)	Corrective Action
(d) Employee alarm system. An employer must have and maintain an employee alarm system. The employee alarm system must use a distinctive signal for each purpose and comply with the requirements in § 1910.165.		
1910.165(a) **Scope and application.** **1910.165(a)(1)** This section applies to all emergency employee alarms installed to meet a particular OSHA standard. This section does not apply to those discharge or supervisory alarms required on various fixed extinguishing systems or to supervisory alarms on fire suppression, alarm or detection systems unless they are intended to be employee alarm systems.		
1910.165(a)(2) The requirements in this section that pertain to maintenance, testing and inspection shall apply to all local fire alarm signaling systems used for alerting employees regardless of the other functions of the system.		
1910.165(a)(3) All pre-discharge employee alarms installed to meet a particular OSHA standard shall meet the requirements of paragraphs (b)(1) through (4), (c), and (d)(1) of this section.		
1910.165(b) **General requirements.** **1910.165(b)(1)** The employee alarm system shall provide warning for necessary emergency action as called for in the emergency action plan, or for reaction time for safe escape of employees from the workplace or the immediate work area, or both.		
1910.165(b)(2) The employee alarm shall be capable of being perceived above ambient noise or light levels by all employees in the affected portions of the workplace. Tactile devices may be used to alert those employees who would not otherwise be able to recognize the audible or visual alarm.		
1910.165(b)(3) The employee alarm shall be distinctive and recognizable as a signal to evacuate the work area or to perform actions designated under the emergency action plan.		
1910.165(b)(4) The employer shall explain to each employee the preferred means of reporting emergencies, such as manual pull box alarms, public address systems, radio or telephones. The employer shall post emergency telephone numbers near telephones, or employee notice boards, and other conspicuous locations when telephones serve as a means of reporting emergencies. Where a communication system also serves as the employee alarm system, all emergency messages shall have priority over all non-emergency messages.		

	Compliance (Yes or No)	Corrective Action
1910.165(b)(5) The employer shall establish procedures for sounding emergency alarms in the workplace. For those employers with 10 or fewer employees in a particular workplace, direct voice communication is an acceptable procedure for sounding the alarm provided all employees can hear the alarm. Such workplaces need not have a back-up system.		
1910.165(c) **Installation and restoration.** **1910.165(c)(1)** The employer shall assure that all devices, components, combinations of devices or systems constructed and installed to comply with this standard are approved. Steam whistles, air horns, strobe lights or similar lighting devices, or tactile devices meeting the requirements of this section are considered to meet this requirement for approval.		
1910.165(c)(2) The employer shall assure that all employee alarm systems are restored to normal operating condition as promptly as possible after each test or alarm. Spare alarm devices and components subject to wear or destruction shall be available in sufficient quantities and locations for prompt restoration of the system.		
1910.165(d) **Maintenance and testing.** **1910.165(d)(1)** The employer shall assure that all employee alarm systems are maintained in operating condition except when undergoing repairs or maintenance.		
1910.165(d)(2) The employer shall assure that a test of the reliability and adequacy of non-supervised employee alarm systems is made every two months. A different actuation device shall be used in each test of a multi-actuation device system so that no individual device is used for two consecutive tests.		
1910.165(d)(3) The employer shall maintain or replace power supplies as often as is necessary to assure a fully operational condition. Back-up means of alarm, such as employee runners or telephones, shall be provided when systems are out of service.		
1910.165(d)(4) The employer shall assure that employee alarm circuitry installed after January 1, 1981, which is capable of being supervised is supervised and that it will provide positive notification to assigned personnel whenever a deficiency exists in the system. The employer shall assure that all supervised employee alarm systems are tested at least annually for reliability and adequacy.		

	Compliance (Yes or No)	Corrective Action
1910.165(d)(5) The employer shall assure that the servicing, maintenance and testing of employee alarms are done by persons trained in the designed operation and functions necessary for reliable and safe operation of the system.		
1910.165(e) Manual operation. The employer shall assure that manually operated actuation devices for use in conjunction with employee alarms are unobstructed, conspicuous and readily accessible.		
(e)Training. An employer must designate and train employees to assist in a safe and orderly evacuation of other employees.		
(f)Review of emergency action plan. An employer must review the emergency action plan with each employee covered by the plan: (1)When the plan is developed or the employee is assigned initially to a job; (2)When the employee's responsibilities under the plan change; and (3)When the plan is changed.		

Source: OSHA.

Elements of an Emergency Action Plan

OSHA 1910.38 for Emergency Action Plans

Part Number: 1910   **Title:** Emergency Action Plans

Part Title: Occupational Safety and Health Standards

Subpart: E

Subpart Title: Means of Egress

Standard Number: 1910.38

1910.38(a) *Application.* An employer must have an emergency action plan whenever an OSHA standard in this part requires one. The requirements in this section apply to each such emergency action plan.

1910.38(b) *Written and oral emergency action plans.* An emergency action plan must be in writing, kept in the workplace, and available to employees for review. However, an employer with 10 or fewer employees may communicate the plan orally to employees.

1910.38(c) Minimum elements of an emergency action plan. An emergency action plan must include at a minimum:

1910.38(c)(1) Procedures for reporting a fire or other emergency;

1910.38(c)(2) Procedures for emergency evacuation, including type of evacuation and exit route assignments;

1910.38(c)(3) Procedures to be followed by employees who remain to operate critical plant operations before they evacuate;

1910.38(c)(4) Procedures to account for all employees after evacuation;

1910.38(c)(5) Procedures to be followed by employees performing rescue or medical duties; and

1910.38(c)(6) The name or job title of every employee who may be contacted by employees who need more information about the plan or an explanation of their duties under the plan.

1910.38(d) Employee alarm system. An employer must have and maintain an employee alarm system. The employee alarm system must use a distinctive signal for each purpose and comply with the requirements in § 1910.165.

1910.38(e) Training. An employer must designate and train employees to assist in a safe and orderly evacuation of other employees.

1910.38(f) Review of emergency action plan. An employer must review the emergency action plan with each employee covered by the plan: 1910.38(f)(1) When the plan is developed or the employee is assigned initially to a job;

1910.38(f)(2) When the employee's responsibilities under the plan change; and 1910.38(f)(3) When the plan is changed.

[45 FR 60703, Sept. 12, 1980; FR 67 67963, Nov. 7, 2002]

Source. OSHA.

Elements of a Fire Prevention Plan

<table>
<tr><td colspan="2">OSHA 1910.39 Fire Prevention Plans</td></tr>
<tr><td colspan="2">

Part Number: 1910   **Title:** Fire Prevention Plans

Part Title: Occupational Safety and Health Standards

Subpart: E

Subpart Title: Means of Egress

Standard Number: 1910.39

1910.39(a) Application. An employer must have a fire prevention plan when an OSHA standard in this part requires one. The requirements in this section apply to each such fire prevention plan.

1910.39(b)   Written and oral fire prevention plans. A fire prevention plan must be in writing, be kept in the workplace, and be made available to employees for review. However, an employer with 10 or fewer employees may communicate the plan orally to employees.

1910.39(c) Minimum elements of a fire prevention plan. A fire prevention plan must include:

1910.39(c)(1) A list of all major fire hazards, proper handling and storage procedures for hazardous materials, potential ignition sources and their control, and the type of fire protection equipment necessary to control each major hazard;

1910.39(c)(2) Procedures to control accumulations of flammable and combustible waste materials;

1910.39(c)(3) Procedures for regular maintenance of safeguards installed on heat-producing equipment to prevent the accidental ignition of combustible materials;

1910.39(c)(4) The name or job title of employees responsible for maintaining equipment to prevent or control sources of ignition or fires; and

1910.39(c)(5) The name or job title of employees responsible for the control of fuel source hazards.

1910.39(d) Employee information. An employer must inform employees upon initial assignment to a job of the fire hazards to which they are exposed. An employer must also review with each employee those parts of the fire prevention plan necessary for self-protection.

[FR 67 67963, Nov. 7, 2002]

</td></tr>
</table>

Source: OSHA.

FEMA RESOURCES

Agency Overview

The Federal Emergency Management Agency (FEMA) is part of the U.S. Department of Homeland Security (DHS). FEMA's mission is as follows:

> *…to support our citizens and first responders to ensure that as a nation we work together to build sustain, and improve our capacity to prepare, protect against, respond to, recover from, and mitigate all hazards. (www.fema.gov/about)*

The Robert T. Stafford Disaster Relief and Emergency Assistance Act, PL 100-707 was signed into law November 23, 1988 and amended the Disaster Relief Act of 1974, PL 93-288. This Act constitutes the statutory authority for most federal disaster response activities especially as they pertain to FEMA and FEMA programs. FEMA has more than 3,700 full-time employees working at FEMA headquarters in Washington D.C., at regional and area offices across the country, at the Mount Weather Emergency Operations Center, and at the National Emergency Training Center in Emmitsburg, Maryland. FEMA also has nearly 4,000 standby disaster assistance employees who are available for deployment after disasters.

Often FEMA works in partnership with other organizations that are part of the nation's emergency management system. These partners include state and local emergency management agencies, 27 federal agencies, and the American Red Cross. FEMA offices and contacts are listed below and can be accessed online at the following links:

Offices and contacts
http://www.fema.gov/about/regions/regioni/index.shtm

- Center for Faith Based and Neighborhood Partnerships
- Office of Chief Financial Officer
- Office of Disability Integration and Coordination
- Office of Equal Rights
- Office of the Executive Secretariat
- Office of External Affairs (includes Disaster Operations, Intergovernmental Affairs, International Affairs, Legislative Affairs, Private Sector Outreach, and Public Affairs
- Resource Management and Administration)
- Office of Chief Counsel
- Office of Federal Coordinating Officer Operations
- Office of Policy and Programs Analysis
- Defense Production Act Program Division

OSHA regional offices: http://www.fema.gov/about/regions/regioni/index.shtm
- Region I (Connecticut, Maine, Massachusetts, New Hampshire, Rhode Island, Vermont)
- Region II (New Jersey, New York, Puerto Rico, and the Virgin Islands)

- <u>Region III</u> (Delaware, District of Columbia, Maryland, Pennsylvania, Virginia and W. Virginia)

- <u>Region IV</u> (Alabama, Florida, Georgia, Kentucky, Mississippi, N. Carolina, S. Carolina and Tennessee)

- <u>Region V</u> (Illinois, Indiana, Michigan, Minnesota, Ohio and Wisconsin)

- <u>Region VI</u> (Arkansas, Louisiana, New Mexico, Oklahoma and Texas)

- <u>Region VII</u> (Iowa, Kansas, Missouri and Nebraska)

- <u>Region VIII</u> (Colorado, Montana, N. Dakota, S. Dakota, Utah and Wyoming)

- <u>Region IX</u> (Arizona, California, Hawaii, Nevada, American Samoa, Guam, Commonwealth of the Northern Mariana Islands, Republic of the Marshall Islands, and Federated States of Micronesia)

- <u>Region X</u> (Alaska, Idaho, Oregon and Washington)

Family Emergency Planning

Your family may not be together when disaster strikes, so it is important to plan in advance. Plan for how you will contact one another; how you will get back together; and what you will do depending on different situations. Commit a weekend to updating telephone numbers, buying emergency supplies, and reviewing your emergency plan as a family. In addition, consider the following:

- Identify an out-of town contact. It may be easier to make a long-distance phone call than to call across town, so an out-of-town contact may be in a better position to communicate among separated family members.

- Be sure every member of your family knows the phone number and has a cell phone, coins, or a prepaid phone card to call the emergency contact. If you have a cell phone, program that person(s) as "ICE" (In Case of Emergency) in your phone. If you are in an accident, emergency personnel will often check your ICE listings to contact someone you know. Make sure to tell your family and friends you've listed them as emergency contacts.

- Teach family members how to use text messaging (also knows as SMS or Short Message Service). Text messages can often get around network disruptions when a phone call might not be able to get through.

- Subscribe to alert services. Many communities now have systems that will send instant text alerts or e-mails to let you know about inclement weather, road closings, local emergencies, and so forth. Sign up by visiting your <u>local Office of Emergency Management web site</u>.

Planning to Stay or Go

Depending on your circumstances and the nature of the emergency, the first important decision is whether you stay where you are or evacuate. Understand and plan for both possibilities. Use common sense and available information, including what you are learning here, to determine if there is an immediate danger. In any emergency, local authorities may or may not immediately be able to provide information on what is happening and what you should do. However, you should watch TV, listen to the radio, or check the Internet often for information or official instruction as it becomes available.

Emergency Plans

Use the New Online Family Emergency Planning Tool created by the Ready Campaign in conjunction with the Ad Council to prepare a <u>printable Comprehensive Family Emergency Plan</u>. Use the <u>Quick Share application</u> to help your family in assembling a quick reference list of contact information for your family, and a meeting place for emergency situations. You may also want to inquire about emergency plans at places where your family spends time: work, daycare, and school. If no plans exist, consider volunteering to help create one. Talk to your neighbors about how you can work together in the event of an emergency. You will be better prepared to safely reunite your family and loved ones during an emergency if you think ahead and communicate with others in advance. Read more at <u>School and Workplace</u>.

Information

Find out what kinds of disasters, both natural and man-made, are most likely to occur in your area and how you will be notified. Methods of getting your attention vary from community to community. One common method is to broadcast via emergency radio and TV broadcasts. You might hear a special siren, or get a telephone call, or emergency workers may go door-to-door (<u>www.ready.gov</u>).

Basics of Survival

When preparing for a possible emergency, it is best to think first about the basics of survival. Visit <u>http://www.ready.gov/america/getakit/</u> for more information on preparing a survival kit and review each of the following lists for suggestions:

Recommended Items to Include in a Basic Emergency Supply Kit:

- **One gallon of water per person per day for at least three days, for drinking and sanitation**

- At least a three-day supply of non-perishable food

- Battery-powered or hand crank radio and a NOAA Weather Radio with tone alert and extra batteries for both

- Flashlight and extra batteries

- First-aid kit

- Whistle to signal for help

- Dust mask, to help filter contaminated air and plastic sheeting and duct tape to shelter-in-place

- Moist towelettes, garbage bags, and plastic ties for personal sanitation

- Wrench or pliers to turn off utilities

- Can opener for food (if kit contains canned food)

- Local maps/cell phone with chargers

Additional Items to Consider Adding to an Emergency Supply Kit:

- Prescription medications and eyeglasses

- Infant formula and diapers

- Pet food and extra water for your pet
- Important family documents such as copies of insurance policies, identification and bank account records in a waterproof, portable container
- Cash or traveler's checks and change
- Emergency reference material such as a first-aid book or information from www.ready.gov
- Sleeping bag or warm blanket for each person. Consider additional bedding if you live in a cold-weather climate.
- Complete change of clothing including a long sleeved shirt, long pants and sturdy shoes. Consider additional clothing if you live in a cold-weather climate.
- Household chlorine bleach and medicine dropper (when diluted nine parts water to one part bleach, bleach can be used as a disinfectant. Or in an emergency, you can use it to treat water by using 16 drops of regular household liquid bleach per gallon of water. Do not use scented, color-safe, or bleaches with added cleaners.
- Fire extinguisher/matches in a waterproof container.
- Feminine supplies and personal hygiene items.
- Mess kits, paper cups, plates and plastic utensils, paper towels.
- Paper and pencil/books, games, puzzles, or other activities for children (www.ready.gov).

Independent Study Programs for Distant Learning

The Emergency Management Institute (EMI) offers free, self-paced courses designed for people who have emergency management responsibilities and the general public. All are offered free-of-charge to those who qualify for enrollment. To get a complete listing of courses visit http://www.training.fema.gov/IS/. FEMA's Independent Study Program offers courses that support the nine mission areas identified by the National Preparedness Goal as listed below:

- Incident Management
- Operational Planning
- Disaster Logistics
- Emergency Communications
- Service to Disaster Victims
- Continuity Programs
- Public Disaster Communications
- Integrated Preparedness
- Hazard Mitigation

Use of Social Media

FEMA has been engaging in Web 2.0 tools and on social media sites nationwide as part of its mission to prepare the nation for disasters. FEMA's goals with social media are: to provide timely and accurate information related to disaster preparedness response and recovery; provide the public with another avenue for insight into the agency's operations; and engage in what has already become a critical medium in today's world of communications. FEMA's social media ventures function as supplemental outreach, and as appropriate channels for unofficial input.

All FEMA social media accounts outside of the www.FEMA.gov domain carry the branded *femainfocus* look and feel. This provides consistency and accountability for content so the public and FEMA partners can be assured the content is authorized and the information is accurate. Citizens can engage more easily with the emergency management community through social media sites, and increase their role in disaster preparedness, response, and recovery.

Starting with YouTube as a platform to host and share videos, FEMA began capturing stories from disaster response and recovery efforts to explain the scope of its mission. Videos have ranged in subject from preparedness, response, and recovery to mitigation and explanations of how specific federal aid programs operate. The subjects, or voices, have been FEMA staff, state and local authorities, and individuals affected by disasters. The approach to these Web videos was to capture the voice and perspective of the community involved in a disaster and present it as an opportunity to help educate others on FEMA's mission and programs.

FEMA has been using Twitter www.twitter.com/femainfocus since October, 2008 as a means to offer information about the agency's mission, efforts, and perspective. The agency also launched its YouTube page www.youtube.com/fema in October, 2008 to provide stories about how its programs work in communities nationwide as they prepare for, respond to, and recover from disasters.

FEMA External Affairs has been pragmatically adapting its communications efforts towards inclusion of social media since June, 2008. In fact, FEMA External Affairs, in coordination with the FEMA Office of Chief Counsel, was one of the first federal agencies to achieve a modified user agreement with Google in May, 2008, providing a working example for other federal agencies. It also broke new ground for a federal agency through its use of Twitter to host the first all-access press conference through the tool. For the Twitter event, FEMA set new ground rules for federal engagement and provided its results online in a move to usher in full transparency www.fema.gov/media/2009/010909.shtm behind federal social media exchanges.

The following is a list of FEMA.gov – based and social media sites that FEMA uses to engage the public.

- RSS Feeds (www.fema.gov/help/rss.shtm) – FEMA currently offers national-level RSS feeds that provide subscribers with automated updated information. Apart from press release and disaster declaration information, subscribers can receive notifications on the issuance of new situation reports and photographs added to the official FEMA Photo Library.

- Widgets (www.fema.gov/help/widgets/) – Widgets provide data feeds through transportable well-defined web-based graphical interfaces.

- Multimedia (www.fema.gov/medialibrary) – The Multimedia site provides contributor an end-user interaction on a .gov platform. This site currently hosts videos, podcasts, photos and text-based documents that are presented in collections related to disasters and subject matter. It permits Web 2.0 functions such as embed coding and sharing.

Below is a list of links for following FEMA's presence on other third party sites for your reference. FEMA does not endorse any non-government Web sites, companies, or applications.

- Youtube (www.youtube.com/fema) – Video service that provides FEMA opportunity to tell timely and accurate stories of its mission. The FEMA channel is used to help state partners host and share public service announcements, explain federal reimbursement process and mitigation efforts local to specific communities. These short videos provide access to the overall operation and offer an opportunity for the voices within the community to explain how programs affect their lives.

- Twitter (www.twitter.com/femainfocus) – Microblog that gives FEMA the opportunity to direct followers and users of the tool to specific information in a timely manner, such as during emergencies and disasters. There is a national Twitter account and there are regional Twitter accounts.

    o National (www.twitter.com/femainfocus)

    o Region I (Connecticut, Maine, Massachusetts, New Hampshire, Rhode Island, Vermont) (www.twitter.com/femaregion1)

    o Region II (New Jersey, New York, Puerto Rico, and the Virgin Islands) (www.twitter.com/femaregion2)

    o Region III (Delaware, District of Columbia, Maryland, Pennsylvania, Virginia and W. Virginia) (www.twitter.com/femaregion3)

    o Region IV (Alabama, Florida, Georgia, Kentucky, Mississippi, N. Carolina, S. Carolina and Tennessee) (www.twitter.com/femaregion4)

    o Region V (Illinois, Indiana, Michigan, Minnesota, Ohio and Wisconsin) (www.twitter.com/femaregion5)

    o Region VI (Arkansas, Louisiana, New Mexico, Oklahoma and Texas) (www.twitter.com/femaregion6)

    o Region VII (Iowa, Kansas, Missouri and Nebraska) (www.twitter.com/femaregion7)

    o Region VIII (Colorado, Montana, N. Dakota, S. Dakota, Utah and Wyoming) (www.twitter.com/femaregion8)

    o Region IX (Arizona, California, Hawaii, Nevada, American Samoa, Guam, Commonwealth of the Northern Mariana Islands, Republic of the Marshall Islands, and Federated States of Micronesia) (www.twitter.com/femaregion9)

    o Region X (Alaska, Idaho, Oregon and Washington) (www.twitter.com/femaregion10)

    o US Fire Administration (www.twitter.com/usfire)

- Facebook (www.facebook.com/fema) – FEMA has been using its FaceBook account since May, 2009 to provide a forum for preparedness information and to engage the public with links and topics.

- Google Books – FEMA has been working with Google Books to provide its published content in a free, easy to access format online. FEMA currently offers publications on preparedness, mitigation and its recovery programs in hard copy through its distribution warehouse.

FEMA will be able to provide this content and future content on a broader scale by leveraging the technology and resources available (www.fema.gov).

Comprehensive Planning Guide (CPG 101)

The FEMA Comprehensive Planning Guide is required for planning by most public-sector agencies. CPG 101 is part of a series of CPGs published by FEMA. CPG 101 discusses the steps used to produce an emergency operations plan (EOP), possible plan structures, and components of a basic plan and its annexes. CPGs provide detailed information about planning considerations for specific functions, hazards, and threats.

CPG 101 is the foundation for state, territorial, tribal, and local emergency planning in the United States. Planners in other disciplines, organizations, and the private sector, as well as other levels of government, may find this Guide useful in the development of their EOPs.

CPG 101 integrates key concepts from national preparedness policies and doctrines, as well as lessons learned from disasters, major incidents, national assessments, and grant programs. CPG 101 provides methods for planners to:

- Conduct community-based planning that engages the whole community by using a planning process that represents the actual population in the community and involves community leaders and the private sector in the planning process

- Ensure plans are developed through an analysis of risk

- Identify operational assumptions and resource demands

- Prioritize plans and planning efforts to support their seamless transition from development to execution for any threat or hazard

- Integrate and synchronize efforts across all levels of government

CPG 101 incorporates the following concepts from operational planning research and day-to-day experience:

- The process of planning is just as important as the resulting document.

- Plans are not scripts followed to the letter, but are flexible and adaptable to the actual situation.

- Effective plans convey the goals and objectives of the intended operation and the actions needed to achieve them.

Successful operations occur when organizations know their roles, understand how they fit into the overall plan, and are able to execute the plan (www.fema.gov).

Voluntary Private Sector Preparedness Accreditation and Certification Program

The Department of Homeland Security Voluntary Private Sector Preparedness Accreditation and Certification Program (PS-Prep) is mandated by Title IX of the *Implementing Recommendations of the 9/11 Commission Act of 2007 (the Act.)* Congress directed the

Department of Homeland Security (DHS) to develop and implement a voluntary program of accreditation and certification of private entities using standards adopted by DHS that promote private sector preparedness, including disaster management, emergency management, and business continuity programs.

The purpose of the PS-Prep Program is to enhance nationwide resilience in an all-hazards environment by encouraging private sector preparedness. The program provides a mechanism by which a private sector entity—a company, facility, not-for-profit corporation, hospital, stadium, university, and so forth,—may be certified by an accredited third party establishing that the private sector entity conforms to one or more preparedness standards adopted by DHS.

Prior to the PS-Prep program, there was no comprehensive set of standards by which American businesses and other private sector entities could assess their preparedness for all hazards. Having a plan to reduce the impact of all hazards on business and protect employees can help ensure that a business is able to recover and reopen following a disaster or other emergencies.

Participation in the PS-Prep program is completely voluntary. No private sector entity will be required by DHS to comply with any standard adopted under the program. However, DHS encourages all private sector entities to seriously consider seeking certification on one or more standards that will be adopted by DHS.

Congress directed DHS to designate one or more standards for assessing private sector preparedness. The standards will be used by accredited certifying entities to evaluate and certify compliance by private sector entities with the standards adopted by DHS.

DHS published a notice in the Federal Register in Oct. 2009, announcing its intent to adopt the three standards listed below. Following a series of regional public meetings and the incorporation of public comments, the three standards were approved in June 2010, based on scalability, balance of interest and relevance to PS-Prep:

- ASIS International SPC.1-2009 *Organizational Resilience: Security Preparedness, and Continuity Management System – Requirements with Guidance for use (2009 Edition).* Available at no cost.

- British Standards Institution 25999 *(2007 Edition) – Business Continuity Management.(BS 25999:2006-1 Code of practice for business continuity management and BS 25999: 2007-2 Specification for business continuity management)* The British Standards Institution is making both parts available for a reduced fee of $19.99 each.

- National Fire Protection Association 1600-*Standard on Disaster / Emergency Management and Business Continuity Programs, 2007 and 2010 editions.* Available at no cost.

Each of these standards comprehensively deals with preparedness and can be applied to the majority of private sector entities.

DHS will continue to accept comments on PS-Prep, the three adopted standards, and/or proposals to adopt any other similar standard that satisfies the target criteria of the December 2008 Federal Register notice which announced the program. DHS will review any comments received or proposals for DHS adoption of additional standards and, when merited, will publish a Federal Register notice providing the results of that review or notifying the public of an intention to adopt additional standards.

Small Business Considerations

The Act recognizes that small businesses need to be treated differently in the PS-Prep program, and requires DHS to give special consideration to small business concerns (as defined by Section 3 of the Small Business Act (15 U.S.C. 632)). The December 24, 2008, Federal Register Notice (73 FR 79140) contained an extensive discussion of DHS' approaches to best reflect the interests of small businesses and the purpose of the PS-Prep Program. DHS continues to seek comments from small businesses and others on the adoption of these standards and their impact on future decisions to seek certification under the PS-Prep Program.

Understanding the Process

Certification, in the context of this program, is confirmation that an accredited third party certification organization has validated a private sector entity's preparedness to a standard. Once an organization is certified, there will be a periodic reassessment and audit process so the certification organization can continue to have confidence in the organization's conformity to emergency preparedness and business continuity management system. The certifying organizations will be accredited by ANAB. DHS will maintain and make public a listing of any private sector entity certified as being in compliance with PS-Prep, if that private sector entity consents to such listing.

Program Monitoring

DHS monitors the effectiveness of the program on an ongoing basis, and reviews the accreditation and certification program annually to ensure its effectiveness, and to include the operations and management of any of the accreditation and certification bodies and the designated standards. DHS makes improvements and adjustments to PS-Prep as necessary and appropriate.

How to Get Involved

Private sector entities can get involved in PS-Prep by submitting comments on the identified standards, suggesting additional private sector standards to be adopted by DHS, and participating in future public meetings on the topic. More details can be obtained by visiting the Web site at: http://www.fema.gov/media/fact_sheets/vpsp.shtm

FEMA Tribal Policy

In response to increasing nation-to-nation relationship building efforts with tribal communities worldwide, the Department of Homeland Security (DHS) announced an initiative for increased consultation and coordination with federally recognized tribes across the United States to protect the safety and security of all individuals on tribal lands through the DHS Tribal Consultation and Coordination Plan. As a result, and in support of the Obama Administration and the DHS' effort, FEMA engaged all federally-recognized tribes to gather suggested revisions to FEMA's existing Tribal Policy. This revised policy statement was based on feedback received, to enhance FEMA's relationship with the Nation's American Indian and Alaska Native Tribal communities to support preparing for, recovering from, mitigating, and responding to all natural and man-made hazards and disasters.

FEMA's policy, as first stated in the September 25, 1998 FEMA Tribal Policy, applies to the American Indian and Alaska Native Tribal Governments as follows:

> *In the spirit of community, FEMA commits itself to building a strong and lasting partnership with American Indians and Alaska Natives to assist them in preparing for the hazards they face, reducing their disaster vulnerabilities, responding quickly and effectively when disasters strike, and recovering in their aftermath.*

This policy applies to all disasters declared after publication of this document. It is intended to guide all personnel responsible for engaging in consultation and coordination with federally-recognized tribal communities across the United States.

FEMA recognizes that the participation of American Indian and Alaska Native Tribal Governments is vital to enhancing nation-to-nation relations and will continue to seek their consultation. FEMA is committed to enhancing the implementation of this policy by working more closely with our governmental partners in the Nation's American Indian and Alaskan Native Tribal communities with the publication of the revised policy. FEMA echos the sentiment expressed by U.S. Secretary Napolitano that this partnership will lead to "better policy outcomes" and will ultimately assist FEMA in achieving its mission.

FEMA also recognizes the need to support the unique status of the American Indian and Alaska Native Tribal governments by engaging in meaningful dialogue when developing and implementing policy directives that will assist the tribal community with their emergency management needs that fall under the auspices of FEMA. This includes, but is not limited to, the building, sustaining, and improvement of tribal capability to prepare for, protect against, respond to, recover from, and mitigate all hazards.

This policy outlines the guiding principles and establishes implementation objectives under which all employees of FEMA are to operate with regard to Federally-recognized American Indian and Alaska Native Tribal governments.

In addition, FEMA acknowledges the inherent sovereignty of American Indian and Alaska Native Tribal governments, the trust responsibility of the federal government, and the nation-to-nation relationship between the U.S. Government and American Indian and Alaska Native Tribal governments as established by specific statutes, treaties, court decisions, executive orders, regulations, and policies. FEMA further acknowledges the precedents of the Constitution, the President of the United States, and the U.S. Congress as the foundation of this policy's content.

This policy is intended to be flexible and practical providing for the evolution of partnerships among FEMA, American Indian and Alaska Native Tribal governments, state and local governments, and other federal agencies. Working within existing statutes and authorities, FEMA will strive to be consistent in the Agency's interactions with American Indian and Alaska Native Tribal governments nationwide.

This policy is consistent with existing law and does not alter or supersede the authorities of FEMA or those of any other Federal agencies. Further, the policy does not diminish or modify existing Tribal government authority in any way, nor does it suggest recognition of Tribal authority that does not currently exist beyond inherent tribal sovereignty. FEMA has authority to work with American Indian and Alaska Native Tribal governments under existing law.

FEMA will examine the feasibility of strengthening the nation-to-nation relationship with Tribal nations in the following areas:

- Review portions of the Robert T. Stafford Disaster Relief & Emergency Assistance Act, other laws, policies, and administrative rules in emergency management activities to determine how that may allow FEMA to work more directly with local tribal communities.

- FEMA will encourage states to incorporate the inclusion of tribal governments into grant programs and processes to support the trust responsibility between the government and nation-to-nation relationship.

- Consider the designation of full-time tribal liaisons in appropriate FEMA regional offices and explore the possibility of assigning attorneys within the FEMA Office of Chief Counsel (OCC) who are trained and experienced in Federal Indian Law.

- Send senior FEMA leadership periodically to engage tribal government leadership in planning discussions prior to disasters and coordinate follow-up visits to discuss practical solutions.

- Consider expanding existing training efforts to include the development and delivery of regional homeland security and emergency management training to tribal locations (on-site)

For more information on FEMA's Tribal Policy visit the Web site at http://www.fema.gov/government/tribal/natamerpolcy.shtm. The current policy supersedes the FEMA Tribal Policy published in the Federal Register – January 12, 1999 and all previous guidance on this subject. This policy does not automatically expire, but is reviewed every three years from the date of publication (www.fema.gov).

References

Centers for Disease Control and Prevention (CDC). Radiation Studies Branch (RSB), Division of Environmental Hazards and Health Effects (EHHE), National Center for Environmental Health (NCEH), Coordinating Center for Environmental Health and Injury Prevention (CCEHIP), CDC Radiation Emergencies/Dirty Bombs. *CDC Emergency Preparedness & Response Site*. Center of Disease Control and Prevention, downloaded April 7, 2011 from http://emergency.cdc.gov/radiation/dirtybombs.asp.

Comprehensive Planning Guide (CPG 101). *http://www.fema.gov*. FEMA, 1 Nov. 2010. Downloaded April 4, 2011 from http://www.fema.gov/pdf/about/divisions/npd/CPG_101_V2.pdf.

Emergency Management Institute – FEMA Independent Study Program. *National Preparedness Directorate National Training and Education Portal*. n.p., 17 Feb. 2011. Downloaded April 4, 2011 from http://www.training.fema.gov/IS/.

FEMA. About FEMA. *Federal Emergency Management Agency.* FEMA, 22 Mar. 2011. Downloaded April 3, 2011 from http://www.fema.gov/about/.

FEMA. FEMA Tribal Policy. *FEMA Federal Emergency Management Agency.* FEMA, 29 June 2010. Downloaded April 4, 2011 from http://www.fema.gov/government/tribal/natamerpolcy.shtm.

FEMA. Use of Social Media Tools at FEMA. *FEMA Federal Emergency Management Agency.* Version Release Number: FNF-09-040. FEMA, 6 Nov. 2009. Downloaded April 4, 2011 from http://www.fema.gov/news/newsrelease.fema?id=49302.

FEMA. Region I. FEMA. *Federal Emergency Management Agency.* n.p., 1 Apr. 2011. Downloaded April 3, 2011 from http://www.fema.gov/about/regions/regioni/index.shtm.

FEMA. Voluntary Private Sector Preparedness Accreditation and Certification Program. *FEMA Federal Emergency Management Agency.* n.p., 11 Aug. 2010. Downloaded April 4, 2011 from http://www.fema.gov/media/fact_sheets/vpsp.shtm.

OSHA. Homeland Security: Evacuation Planning Matrix. *Occupational Safety and Health Administration – Home.* OSHA, 8 May 2003. Downloaded April 7, 2011 from http://www.osha.gov/dep/evacmatrix/index.html.

Ready.gov. Get A Kit. *Ready.gov – Prepare. Plan. Stay Informed.* n.p., 10 Nov. 2010. Downloaded April 3, 2011 from http://www.ready.gov/america/getakit/.

Ready.gov. Make a Family Communications Plan. *Ready.gov – Prepare. Plan. Stay Informed.* FEMA, n.d. Downloaded April 7, 2011 from http://www.ready.gov/america/makeaplan/.

SECTION IV-C
ADDITIONAL ONLINE RESOURCES

[To the Emergency Planner: To access the links in this section, 1. Place the cursor on the topic. 2. Press control and at the same time left click. 3. If the link fails to open, go directly to the source agency to conduct your search.]

- Environmental Protection Agency (EPA) Links

    - Data Bases and Tools

    - Resource Overview for Hazardous Event Response

    - Emergency "A through Z Index" Links

    - Agency Contacts and Resources

- Centers for Disease Control and Prevention (CDC) Links

    - Preparedness and Response Web sites: A to Z

- Other Useful Web sites

ENVIRONMENTAL PROTECTION AGENCY (EPA) LINKS

EPA Databases and Tools

The Environmental Protection Agency (EPA) maintains and makes available resources for emergency planning and responding to events that involve chemical release or exposures. The following list provides databases and tools from the EPA Web site (http://www.epa. gov/emergencies/index.htm). These resources are designed to assist facilities in complying with emergency management regulations, help first responders address emergency situations, improve safety, and provide the public with an increased understanding of chemicals in the community.

EPA Resource Overview for Hazardous Event Response

ALOHA® (Area Locations of Hazardous Atmospheres), part of the CAMEO (Computer-Aided Management of Emergency Operations) suite, is an atmospheric dispersion model used for evaluating releases of hazardous chemical vapors, including toxic gas clouds, fires, and explosions. Using input about the release, ALOHA generates a threat zone estimate. A threat zone is the area where a hazard (toxicity, flammability, thermal radiation, or damaging overpressure) is predicted to exceed a user-specified level of concern. Threat zones can also be plotted on maps with MARPLOT (Mapping Applications for Response, Planning, and Local Operational Tasks) to display the location of facilities storing hazardous materials and vulnerable locations (such as hospitals and schools). Specific information about these locations can be extracted from CAMEO information modules to help make decisions about the degree of hazard posed. For more information: Downloading, Installing, and Running ALOHA.

ARIP (Accidental Release Information Program)

The Accidental Release Information Program (ARIP) database (July, 1999) (ZIP) (4 files, 1.1MB) is contained in a zip file that contains the ARIP database file (DBF format) and supporting documentation.

CAMEO (Computer-Aided Management of Emergency Operations)

The CAMEO software suite consists of four core programs: CAMEO, CAMEO Chemicals, MARPLOT, and ALOHA. These programs can be used together or separately. When the programs are used together, they interact seamlessly and information can be linked easily between them. The CAMEO program is a database application that includes several modules (such as Contacts, Facilities, and Resources) to assist with data management requirements under the Emergency Planning and Community Right-to-Know Act (EPCRA). For example, people can use the Facilities and Chemicals in Inventory modules in CAMEO to store Tier II information about the chemical facilities in their communities. CAMEO can also be used to navigate between ALOHA, MARPLOT, and the downloadable version of CAMEO Chemicals. For more information, see the CAMEO homepage and Downloading, Installing, and Running CAMEO.

CAMEO Chemicals

Part of the CAMEO suite, CAMEO Chemicals is a program that allows users to search for chemicals in the CAMEO chemical database, print customized reports with response recommendations, and find out how chemicals would react if they mixed. This program is available as a Web site: http://cameochemicals.noaa.gov/ and also as a downloadable program; however, only the downloadable version can share information with other programs in the suite. For more information (or to get the downloadable version), see the CAMEO Chemicals website.

CERCLIS (Comprehensive Environmental Response, Compensation and Liability Information System)

CERCLIS, or the Comprehensive Environmental Response, Compensation and Liability Information System, contains information on hazardous waste sites, potentially hazardous waste sites, and remedial activities across the nation. The database includes sites that are on the National Priorities List (NPL) or being considered for the NPL. For more information, see CERCLIS Database.

CRW (Chemical Reactivity Worksheet)

The Chemical Reactivity Worksheet (CRW) is a free program that allows users to investigate the reactivity of substances or mixtures of substances. CRW includes a database of reactivity information for more than 5,000 common hazardous chemicals and offers a way to virtually "mix" chemicals—as well as water—to discover what chemical combinations are reactive. CRW also allows users to build a "Custom Chemical Database" containing all the unique materials that are present at a particular facility. CRW has been upgraded by NOAA to include a new FileMaker Runtime user interface, which makes it compatible with the latest computer operating systems. For more information, see Chemical Reactivity Worksheet.

LandView

LandView® is a DVD and CD-ROM publication of data and maps, jointly issued by the Census Bureau, EPA, United States Geological Survey (USGS), and National Oceanic and Atmospheric Administration (NOAA). For more information, see the Official LandView web site at Census Bureau.

MARPLOT (Mapping Applications for Response, Planning, and Local Operational Tasks)

Part of the CAMEO suite, MARPLOT® is a mapping application that people can use to quickly create, view, and modify maps. Users can create their own objects in MARPLOT (e.g., facilities, schools, response assets) and display them on top of a basemap. (There are three basemaps to choose from: standard map files, aerial photos, and topographical maps.) Users can also link objects they have created in MARPLOT to the CAMEO database to store additional information about the objects. For example, users might create an object for a chemical facility in MARPLOT, and then link it to the facility record in CAMEO to quickly get information about the facility's chemical inventory during an emergency response. For more information, see Downloading, Installing, and Running MARPLOT.

National Response Center (NRC)

The National Response Center (NRC), the federal government's national communications center, is staffed 24 hours a day by U.S. Coast Guard officers and marine science technicians and serves as the sole federal point of contact for reporting all hazardous substances and oil spills.

The NRC maintains reports of all releases and spills in a national database. To access this information, see the <u>National Response Center: Data Query Page</u>.

RMP*Comp

RMP*Comp is an electronic tool used to perform the off-site consequence analysis required under the Risk Management Program rule published by the Environmental Protection Agency on July 20, 1996, which implements Section 112(r) of the Clean Air Act. Previously, EPA has referred to this tool as RMP Calculator or RMP Assistant. RMP*Comp makes the same calculations you can make manually by following the procedures described in EPA's guidance document, <u>RMP Offsite Consequence Analysis Guidance (April 1999)</u>. For more information, see <u>RMP*Comp</u>.

RMP*eSubmit

RMP*eSubmit is software for facilities to use in submitting Risk Management Plans (RMPs) required under the Risk Management Program. EPA asks that all facilities use this new method to submit RMPs because it is easy to use, will improve data quality, and will enable users to access RMP 24 hours a day, 7 days a week. Facilities submitting Confidential Business Information (CBI) and Trade Secrets cannot use RMP*eSubmit at this time and must submit using RMP*Submit 2004. For more information, see <u>RMP*eSubmit</u>.

Tier2 Submit

EPA developed Tier2 Submit to help facilities prepare an electronic chemical inventory report. Many states accept Tier2 Submit. For more information, see <u>Tier II Chemical Inventory Reports / Tier2 Submit</u>.

Title III Consolidated List of Lists — May 2010 Version

The Consolidated List of Chemicals Subject to the Emergency Planning and Community Right-to-Know Act (EPCRA) and Section 112(r) of the Clean Air Act (also known as the List of Lists) was prepared to help firms handling chemicals determine whether they need to submit reports under sections 302, 304, or 313 of EPCRA and, for a specific chemical, what reports may need to be submitted. It will also help firms determine whether they will be subject to accident prevention regulations under CAA section 112(r). These lists should be used as a reference tool, not as a definitive source of compliance information. Compliance information for EPCRA is published in the Code of Federal Regulations (CFR), 40 CFR Parts 302, 355, and 372. Compliance information for CAA section 112(r) is published in 40 CFR Part 68. The List of Lists is available several formats.

- <u>Adobe PDF – Title III Consolidated List of Lists – May 2010</u> (105 pp, 497KB, <u>About PDF</u>)

- <u>Microsoft Excel – Title III Consolidated List of Lists – May 2010</u> (296KB, XLS)

Vulnerable Zone Indicator System (VZIS)

VZIS is used to determine whether an address may be in the vulnerable zone of a facility that submitted a Risk Management Plan. For more information, see <u>Vulnerable Zone Indicator System</u>.

Key Links

The EPA programs in the following list ensure preparedness steps to prevent oil spills, chemical accidents, and other events. When these events do occur the mandated response plans are activated.

- <u>Environmental Response Laboratory Network (ERLN)</u>. EPA's National Network of laboratories that can be accessed as needed to support large-scale environmental responses.

- <u>Emergency Planning and Community Right-to-Know Act (EPCRA) Requirements</u>. These requirements help communities prepare for and respond to chemical accidents by requiring facilities to report chemical storage and release information and communities to develop emergency response plans.

- <u>Emergency Response and Cleanup Actions</u>. The EPA coordinates and implements a wide range of activities to ensure that adequate and timely response measures are taken in communities affected by hazardous substances and oil releases.

- <u>Facility Response Plan (FRP) Rule</u>. As part of the Oil Pollution Prevention regulation, some facilities that store and use oil must prepare and submit plans to respond to a worst-case discharge of oil and to a substantial threat of such a discharge.

- <u>Local Governments Reimbursement (LGR) Program</u>. This EPA program helps local governments pay for emergency response measures.

- <u>National Contingency Plan (NCP) Subpart J Product Schedule</u>. Subpart J provides for a schedule of dispersants, other chemicals, and other spill-mitigating devices and substances that may be authorized for use on oil discharges.

- <u>Reporting Oil Discharges and Hazardous Substance Releases</u>. Regulated facilities must report discharges of oil or releases of hazardous substances to EPA, other federal agencies, and/or state and local government agencies.

- <u>Risk Management Plan (RMP)</u>. Facilities that produce, handle, process, distribute, or store certain chemicals must develop and report to EPA an accident prevention plan including a hazard assessment, a prevention history, and an emergency response program.

- <u>Spill Prevention, Control, and Countermeasure (SPCC) Rule</u>. As part of the Oil Pollution Prevention regulation, specific facilities must prepare, amend, and implement SPCC Plans.

EPA Emergency Links

A

About Us

ALOHA: Areal Locations of Hazardous Atmospheres

Alternative Chemical Countermeasures for Oil Spills (NCP Product Schedule - Subpart J)

ARIP: Accidental Release Information Program

B

Basic Information

Bioremediation Agents for Oil Spills

Border Programs

Business Operations Center

C

CAMEO (Computer-Aided Management of Emergency Operations) Web Site

CERCLIS - Comprehensive Environmental Response, Compensation and Liability Information System

Chemical Accident Investigation Reports

Chemical Accident Prevention Provision

Chemicals, Hazardous Substances, and Oil

Chemical Emergency Preparedness and Prevention Advisories

Chemical Safety Alerts

Chemical Safety Audit Reports

Chemical Safety Information, Site Security and Fuels Regulatory Relief Act

Chemical Safety Network

Clean Water Act

Cleanups in My Community

Community Involvement

Contact Us

Criteria for State, Local and Regional Oil Removal Contingency Plans (40 CFR 109)

D

Databases and Tools

Discharge of Oil Regulation

Dispersants for Oil Spills

E

Emergency Management Partners

Emergency Planning and Community Right-to-Know Act (EPCRA) Overview

Emergency Planning and Community Right-to-Know Act (EPCRA) Requirements

Emergency Release Notification Requirements (EPCRA Section 304)

Emergency Response Authorities

Envirofacts Warehouse

Environmental Response Team

EPA Special Teams

Evaluation and Communications Division

F

Facility Response Plan (FRP) Rule

Federal Reading Rooms

Freshwater Spills Symposia

H

Hazardous Chemical Storage Reporting Requirements (EPCRA Sections 311-312)

Hazardous Substances

Hazardous Materials Transportation Act

Hurricane Response

I

Incidents of National Significance (now referred to as Nationally Significant Incidents)

Information Sources

Inter-Agency Teams

International Partnerships and U.S. Border Programs

L

LandView®

Laws and Regulations

Learning Center

List of Lists

Local Emergency Planning Committee (LEPC) Database

Local Emergency Planning Requirements

Local Governments Reimbursement Helpline

Local Governments Reimbursement Program

M

MARPLOT: Mapping Applications for Response, Planning, and Local Operational Tasks

Miscellaneous Oil Spill Control Agents (MOSCA)

Multilateral Programs

N

National Contingency Plan Product Schedule

National Contingency Plan (NCP) Subpart J

National Decontamination Team

National Incident Management System

National Oil and Hazardous Substances Contingency Plan

National Planning and Preparedness Division

National Response Center

National Response Framework (NRF)

National Response System

National Response Team

Nationally Significant Incidents

Newsroom

O

Oil Discharge and Hazardous Substances Release Reporting Requirements

Oil DROP (1997-2003)

Oil Pollution Act

Oil Pollution Prevention Regulation

Oil Program Update (1997-2005)

Oil Update (2007-Present)

On-Scene Coordinators

P

Partners

Policy and Guidance

Preparing for an Emergency

Product Schedule – NCP Subpart J

Programs

Program Operations and Coordination Division

Publications

R

Regional Emergency Management Contacts

Regional Response Teams

Regulation and Policy Development Division

Regulatory and Reporting Information for Government

Reimbursement to Local Governments for Emergency Response To Hazardous Substance Releases Regulation

Report an Environmental Emergency

Reporting Exemptions for Hazardous Substance Releases

Reporting Exemptions for Oil Spills

Response and Clean-up Technologies

Risk Management Program Reporting Center

Risk Management Plan (RMP)

RMP*Comp

RMP*Review

RMP*Submit 2009

S

Science and Research

Small Businesses

Sorbents for Oil Spills

Spill Prevention, Control, and Countermeasure (SPCC) Rule

SPCC Guidance for Regional Inspectors

State Emergency Response Commission (SERC) Contacts

State Environmental Agencies

Subpart J – NCP Product Schedule

Superfund Reportable Quantities (RQs)

Surface Washing Agents for Oil Spills

T

Tier2 Submit

Tier II Chemical Inventory Reports

Title III List of Lists

Tools and Resources for State, Local and Tribal Governments

Toxic Release Inventory

V

Vulnerable Zone Indicator System (VZIS)

W

Where You Live

Window to my Environment

Contacts and Resources

Contact State and Local Environmental Agencies

- Local Emergency Planning Committees (LEPCs)

- State Emergency Response Commissions (SERCs)

- State Environmental Agencies

Contact U.S. EPA

- EPA Office of Emergency Management

- Regional Emergency Management Contacts

How do I...?

Download Tier2*Submit?

Submit a Risk Management Plan?

Apply for local government reimbursement?

Contact EPA emergency management staff?

List a new product on the NCP Product Schedule?

- Border Programs

- CAMEO

- EPCRA

- Facility Response Plan

- Freshwater Spills Symposia

- List of Lists

- Local Governments Reimbursement

- National Response System

- NCP Product Schedule

- Natural Disasters

- Risk Management Plan

- RMP*eSubmit

- SPCC Rule

Learn More About Where You Live

Cleanups in My Community

Find sites where pollution is being or has been cleaned up throughout the United States.

<u>Envirofacts Warehouse</u>
Access several EPA databases with information about environmental activities that may affect air, water, and land anywhere in the United States.

<u>EPA On-Scene Coordinator (OSC) Web Site</u>
Find site-specific information on emergency response and removal actions in each of the 10 EPA regions.

<u>Federal Reading Rooms</u>
Review Risk Management Plan (RMP) information at federal reading rooms.

<u>National Response Center (NRC) Spill Data</u>
Search NRC data for information on reported oil and chemical spills.

<u>Toxic Release Inventory (TRI)</u>
Search information on toxic chemical releases and other waste management activities reported annually by certain covered industry groups as well as federal facilities.

<u>Vulnerable Zone Indicator System (VZIS)</u>
Find out if an address of interest to you—your home, place of work, or your child's school—could be affected by a chemical accident.

<u>Window to my Environment</u>
Enter your zip code to access a wide range of environmental data for an area.

CENTERS FOR DISEASE CONTROL AND PREVENTION (CDC) LINKS

The Centers for Disease Control and Prevention Emergency Preparedness and Response Web site (<u>http://emergency.cdc.gov/</u>) is CDC's primary source of information and resources for preparing for and responding to public health emergencies. This site continues to keep the public informed about public health emergencies and provides the information needed to protect and save lives.

Emergency Preparedness and Response A to Z

A
<u>Abrin</u>

<u>Acids (caustics)</u>

<u>Adamsite (DM)</u>

<u>Americium-241 (Am-241)</u>

<u>Ammonia</u>

Anthrax (*Bacillus anthracis*)

Arenaviruses

Arsenic

Arsine (SA)

Avian Influenza (Bird Flu)

B

Bacillus anthracis (anthrax)

Barium

Benzene

Biotoxins

Bird Flu (Avian Influenza)

Blister agents/vesicants

Blood agents

Botulism (*Clostridium botulinum* toxin)

Brevetoxin

Bromine(CA)

Bromobenzylcyanide(CA)

Brucella species(brucellosis)

Brucellosis (*Brucella* species)

Burkholderia mallei (glanders)

Burkholderia pseudomallei (melioidosis)

BZ

C

Carbon Monoxide

Caustics (acids)

Cesium-137(Cs-137)

Chemical agents

Chlorine (CL)

Chloroacetophenone (CN)

Chlorobenzylidenemalononitrile (CS)

Chloropicrin (PS)

Choking/lung/pulmonary agents

Cholera (*Vibrio cholerae*)

Clostridium botulinum toxin (botulism)

Cobalt-60 (Co-60)

Colchicine

Coxiella burnetii (Q fever)

Cyanide

Cyanogen chloride (CK)

D

Diabetes Care During Natural Disasters & Hazards

Dibenzoxazepine (CR)

Digitalis

Dirty bombs

E

Earthquakes

Ebola virus hemorrhagic fever

E. coli O157:H7 (*Escherichia coli*)

Escherichia coli O157:H7 (*E. coli*)

Ethylene glycol

Explosions

Extreme cold / Extreme heat

F

Fentanyls & other opioids

Fire safety

Floods

Flu

Flu, swine Apr 2009

Food safety threats (e.g., *Salmonella* species, *Escherichia coli* O157:H7, *Shigella*)

Forest fires

Francisella tularensis (tularemia)

G

Glanders (*Burkholderia mallei*)

H

H1N1 Flu

Hurricanes

Hydrazine

Hydrofluoric acid (hydrogen fluoride)

Hydrogen cyanide (AC)

Hydrogen fluoride (hydrofluoric acid)

I-J-K

Incapacitating agents

Influenza

Influenza (flu), swine Apr 2009

Iodine-131 (I-131)

L

Landslides & mudslides

Lassa fever

Lewisite (L, L-1, L-2, L-3)

Long-acting anticoagulant (super warfarin)

Lung/choking/pulmonary agents

M

Marburg virus hemorrhagic fever

Mass trauma

Melamine

Melioidosis (*Burkholderia pseudomallei*)

Mercury

Metals

Methyl Bromide

Methyl Isocyanate

Mudslides & landslides

Mustard gas (H) (sulfur mustard)

N

Natural disasters

Nerve agents

Nicotine

Nitrogen mustard (HN-1, HN-2, HN-3)

Nuclear blasts

O-P-Q

Opioids

Organic solvents

Osmium tetroxide

Pandemic Influenza (Flu)

Paraquat

Phosgene(CG)

Phosgene oxime (CX)

Phosphine

Phosphorus, elemental, white or yellow Plague (*Yersinia pestis*)

Plutonium-239 (Pu-239)

Potassium cyanide (KCN)

Power outages Pulmonary/choking/lung agents

Q fever (*Coxiella burnetii*)

R

Radiation exposure/radiological emergencies

Radioisotopes (radioactive isotopes)

Radioactive isotopes (radioisotopes)

Ricin toxin from *Ricinus communis* (castor beans)

Riot control agents/tear gas

S

Salmonella species (salmonellosis)

Salmonella typhi (typhoid fever)

Salmonellosis (*Salmonella* species)

Sarin (GB)

Saxitoxin

Selenium

Severe Weather

Shigella (shigellosis)

Shigellosis (*Shigella*)

Smallpox (variola major)

Sodium azide

Sodium cyanide (NaCN)

Sodium Monofluoroacetate

Soman (GD)

Stibine

Strontium-90 (Sr-90)

Strychnine

Sulfuryl Fluoride

Sulfur mustard (H) (mustard gas)

Super warfarin (long-acting anticoagulant)

Swine influenza (flu)

Swine Flu (H1N1)

T

Tabun (GA)

Tear gas/riot control agents

Tetrodotoxin

Thallium

Tornadoes

Toxic alcohols

Trichothecene

Tsunamis

Tularemia (*Francisella tularensis*)

Typhoid fever (*Salmonella* typhi)

U

Unidentified chemical

Uranium-235 (U-235) & uranium-238 (U-238)

V

Variola major (smallpox)

Vesicants/blister agents

Vibrio cholerae (cholera)

Viral hemorrhagic fevers (filoviruses [e.g., Ebola, Marburg] & arenaviruses [e.g., Lassa, Machupo])

Volcanoes

Vomiting agents

VX

W

Water

Water, Bottled

Water, Drinking

Water, Global

Water, Other

Water, Recreational

Water Treatment

Water Treatment, Emergency

Water Treatment, Global

Water Treatment, Wells

Water-Related Diseases

Web-based Injury Statistics Query and Reporting System — see WISQARS Weight, Healthy — see Healthy Weight

Wells

West Nile Virus in the Workplace West Nile Virus Infection

Western Equine Encephalitis Infection

Whipworm Infection [Trichuriasis]

Whitmore's Disease — see Melioidosis

Whooping Cough — see Pertussis

Wide-ranging OnLine Data for Epidemiologic Research, CDC — see CDC WONDER Wildfires

Wildlife, Infections from Winnable Battles

Winter Storms — see Extreme Cold WISEWOMAN

WISQARS [Web-based Injury Statistics Query and Reporting System]

Women and Vaccination

Women Who Have Sex With Women (WSW), Health of — see Lesbian Health Women's Bleeding Disorders Women's Health

Women's Safety and Health Issues at Work

WONDER, CDC — see CDC WONDER

Work Schedules see also Stress, Occupational

Work Schedules: Shift Work and Long Work Hours

Work Zones, Highway Workforce Genomics Competencies

Workplace Health Hazard Evaluations (HHE)

Workplace Safety & Health Workplace Violence

World Trade Center Response

X-Y-Z

Yersinia pestis (plague)

Zoonotic Hookworm

Zoster — see Shingles

OTHER USEFUL WEB SITES

Note: Web sites may change. If the following links do not work, use a search engine to find the Web site using the organization's name.

American Red Cross: www.redcross.org

Chemical Transportation Emergency Center (CHEMTREC): www.chemtrec.org

Federal Emergency Management Agency information and free services: www.fema.gov

School Emergency & Crisis Response Plan Template-Illinois guide to schools for planning. http://www.isbe.state.il.us/safety/guide.htm

National Fire Protection Association: www.nfpa.org

National Organization on Disability: www.nod.org

National Safety Council: www.nsc.org

National Weather Service: www.nws.noaa.gov

National Weather Service National Hurricane Center: http://www.nhc.noaa.gov

National Weather Service Local River and Flood Forecast Offices: http://www.weather.gov

National Weather Service Pacific Tsunami Warning Centers: http://www.prh.noaa.gov/pr/ptwc

National Weather Service River Forecast Centers: http://www.nws.noaa.gov/rivers_tab.html

National Weather Service West Coast and Alaska Tsunami Warning Center: http://wcatwc.arh.noaa.gov

Occupational Safety and Health Administration Standards: www.osha.gov and click on Regulations

U.S. Department of Homeland Security (three sites): www.whitehouse.gov / www.dhs.gov / www.ready.gov

U.S. Department of Transportation: www.dot.gov

U.S. Environmental Protection Agency: www.epa.gov/enviro

Agency: An agency is a division of government with a specific function, or a nongovernmental organization (e.g., private contractor, business, etc.) that offers a particular kind of assistance. In Incident Command System (ICS), agencies are defined as jurisdictional (having statutory responsibility for incident mitigation), or assisting and/or cooperating (providing resources and/or assistance).

Assessment (pre- and post-disaster) (sometimes referred to as Hazard, Risk, Damage, or Needs Assessment): The process of determining the impact of a potential or real disaster or event on society. It addresses the need for preparedness to prevent or mitigate the potential event, and/or immediate, emergency measures to save and sustain the lives of survivors, and the possibilities for expediting recovery and development. Assessment is an interdisciplinary process undertaken in phases and involving data gathering surveys and the collation, evaluation, and interpretation of information from various sources concerning both direct and indirect estimated and/or real losses, short- and long-term effects. It involves determining what could happen and/or what has happened and what assistance might be needed, but also defining objectives and how relevant assistance can actually be provided to the victims. It requires attention to both short-term needs and long-term implications.

Assistance: The provision on a humanitarian basis of material aid and services necessary to enable people to meet their basic needs for shelter, clothing, water, and food. Assistance is available for extended periods, unlike relief supplies and services that are provided, free of charge, in the period immediately following a crisis.

Buddy System: A means of pairing up or organizing workers to work as a team usually in pairs where each is to look out for the well-being of the other team member as they perform their assigned tasks.

Chemtrec: The Chemical Transportation Emergency Center is a service of the American Chemistry Council. It provides a 24-hour, seven-days-a-week technical information service on chemicals that could be involved in emergencies throughout the United States and elsewhere.

Chronic Exposure: A long duration of time in a contaminant atmosphere or repeated exposures to the contaminant that can cause adverse health effects. These adverse health effects usually manifest themselves after a long period of time from multiple exposures to the contaminant.

Cold Zone: Represents the outer boundary of an emergency incident and an area of the least potential for contaminant exposure to workers and others. It is generally an area intended to act as a buffer to keep persons not involved in the response away from the incident at a safe distance.

Command: The act of directing and/or controlling resources at an incident by virtue of explicit legal, agency, or delegated authority. It may also refer to the Incident Commander.

Command Post: (See Incident Command Post).

Critical Incident Stress Management (CISM): Critical incident stress is a normal response of a healthy person to an abnormal event. Management is conducted through processes like defusing, debriefing, and demobilization. The process takes a comprehensive, systematic, and multi-component approach.

Critique: A meeting or discussion of the pros and cons of how an emergency response incident was conducted by those who participated in the response. This is an element of the termination process of an emergency response that is conducted at the conclusion of the emergency incident's response efforts.

Decontamination: The process of removing or reducing the level of contaminants on people, tools, supplies, and equipment. It is generally used to remove harmful levels of contaminants that will adversely affect human health or well-being.

Degradation: The destruction of equipment such as chemical protective clothing and monitoring instruments that is caused by chemical or physical decomposition of such equipment or its components.

Emergency Action Plan (EAP): The purpose of an EAP is to facilitate and organize employer and employee actions during workplace emergencies. An EAP is a written document that is required by a particular OSHA standard. The elements of the plan shall include, but are not limited to:

1. Escape procedures and emergency escape route assignments.
2. Procedures to be followed by employees who remain to operate critical plant operations before they evacuate.
3. Procedures to account for all employees after emergency evacuation has been completed.
4. Rescue and medical duties for those employees who are to perform them.
5. Means of reporting fires and other emergencies.
6. Names or job titles of people who can be contacted for further information or explanation of duties under the plan.

OSHA standards that require Emergency Action Plans include:

- Process Safety Management of Highly Hazardous Chemicals—1910.119

- Fixed Extinguishing Systems, General—1910.160

- Fire Detection Systems—1910.164

- Grain Handling—1910.272
- Ethylene Oxide—1910.1047
- Methylenedianiline—1910.1050
- 1,3-Butadiene—1910.1051

Emergency Management: The organized analysis, planning, decision making, assignment, and coordination of available resources to the mitigation of, preparedness for, response to, or recovery from emergencies of any kind, whether man-made or of natural sources.

Emergency Manager: The individual within each jurisdiction who is delegated the day-to-day responsibility for developing, testing, exercising, and revising the emergency operations plan and maintaining all emergency management coordination efforts.

Emergency Operations Center (EOC): A location from which centralized emergency management can be performed, generally by civil government officials (municipal, county, state and federal). EOC facilities are established by an agency or jurisdiction to coordinate the overall agency or jurisdictional response and to provide support for the control or mitigation of an emergency.

Emergency Operations Plan (EOP): A state or local document that describes actions to be taken in the event of natural disasters, technological incidents, or weapons of mass destruction attack. It identifies authorities, relationships, and the actions to be taken by whom, what, when, and where, based on predetermined assumptions, objectives, and existing capabilities.

Emergency Response: Those organized actions taken by trained people to assist in controlling and/or reducing the level of losses and associated human suffering that has or could have resulted from an emergency incident.

Emergency Response Agency: Any organization responding to an emergency, or providing mutual aid support to such an organization, whether in the field, at the scene of an incident, or to an emergency operations center.

Emergency Response Personnel: Personnel involved with an agency's response to an emergency.

Emergency Response Plan: A written document that sets forth the tasks or actions that are to be taken once an emergency incident is reported to have occurred. The emergency response plan will usually contain contingency plans for the various types of emergencies that are anticipated to be encountered.

Fire Prevention Plan (FPP): An FPP is a hazard prevention plan that is to ensure advanced planning for evacuations in fire and other emergencies. An FPP is a written document that is required by a particular OSHA standard. The elements of the plan shall include, but are not limited to:

1. A list of major workplace fire hazards and their proper handling and storage procedures, potential ignition sources, their control procedures, and the type of fire protection equipment or systems that can control a fire.

2. Names or job titles of those responsible for maintenance of equipment and systems installed to prevent or control ignition of fires.

3. Names or job titles of those responsible for control of fuel source hazards.

OSHA standards that require Fire Prevention Plans include:

- Ethylene Oxide—1910.1047

- Methylenedianiline—1910.1050

- 1,3-Butadiene—1910.1051

Five-Point Emergency Response Strategy: This strategy outlines the essential points of each of action plans. Each point needs to be understood by on-site responders and by all employees for effective response to emergencies, and evaluation of the response after an event. The five points include:

- Initial notification and ongoing communications

- Assessment

- Command and coordination

- Protective action

- Parallel action

Full Protective Clothing: Personal protective equipment that fully covers the body from head to foot and includes clothing and a respiratory protective device to prevent or minimize exposure to injury from a contaminant in an emergency response operation.

Hazard Analysis: The identification of the potential for, and the magnitude of, an occurrence of a hazard that can cause an emergency incident. It contains three basic parts: the identification of the hazard, the assessment of the hazard, and the available controls that could impact the given hazard. There are various methodologies that are typically used to perform this work, from relatively unsophisticated methods up to and including very complex methods that involve modeling.

Hazard Assessment: An evaluation to identify the likelihood of a specific hazardous event and its consequences. It is an evaluated process to measure or estimate the consequences of the event if it were to occur.

Hazard Control: Any approach or step that is taken to eliminate, prevent, or minimize a hazard that could lead to an emergency incident or one that could cause an emergency incident to become more severe. The steps that could be taken may be personal protective equipment or administrative controls up to and including engineering approaches.

Hazard Identification: This is the process of identifying the intrinsic properties harmful to humans, to process equipment, and/or to the environment that a material has and/or that an activity or industrial process has.

Hazardous Material: A chemical or substance that is regulated by the U.S. Department of Transportation (DOT) because of its inherent nature of being harmful to the public health and/or the environment. DOT regulates interstate and intrastate commercial transport of these materials.

Hazardous Substance: A chemical or material that is regulated by the EPA and/or OSHA because of its inherent nature of being harmful to humans and/or the environment.

HAZWOPER (Hazardous Waste Operations and Emergency Response): An OSHA standard (29 CFR 1910.120) that was required by the Superfund Amendments and Reauthorization Act (SARA) of 1986.

Hot Zone: This zone represents the area with the greatest degree of threat to individuals working in that area and requires the highest level of personal protection equipment. The area should be clearly marked with banner tape or a satisfactory substitute to indicate to workers the high potential for exposure and thus the greatest level of personal protection.

Incident Action Plan: The plan developed at the field response level, which contains objectives reflecting the overall incident strategy and specific tactical actions, and supporting information for the next on-scene operational period. The plan may be oral or written.

Incident Commander: The individual responsible for the command of all functions at the field or on-scene response level related to the management of the emergency event.

Incident Command Post (ICP): The location at which the primary command functions are executed. The ICP may be collocated in the cold zone with the incident base or other incident facilities.

Incident Command System (ICS): An organized, coordinated approach to the control and management of emergency response operations at the scene of an emergency event.

Incipient Stage Fire: A fire that is in the initial stage or beginning stage and that can be controlled or extinguished by portable fire extinguishers, Class II standpipe, or small hose systems without the need for protective clothing or breathing apparatus.

LEPC (Local Emergency Planning Committee): LEPCs are required by EPA regulations and by SARA Title III. It is the local communities committee, which the state has established, that is used to develop and maintain an emergency response plan covering all types of emergencies that may occur in the community.

Liaison Officer: A governmental agency official sent to another agency or organization to facilitate interagency communications and coordination.

National Contingency Plan (NCP): The general overall emergency planning document that is to be used by the federal agencies of the executive branch in assisting the states with handling emergency incidents that occur within the United States or on its borders. The National

Response Team makes up the membership of the federal agencies that have a role to play in the NCP, and that have created the Federal Regional Response Teams, which are located in the federal regional cities so designated.

National Response Center (NRC): A U.S. Coast Guard-operated communications center that is located in Washington, D.C. It is the location that all inadvertent or accidental spills or releases of reportable quantities or more are to be reported, and it is manned 24 hours a day, seven days a week.

National Response Team (NRT): Federal cabinet-level agencies and selected independent federal agencies within the federal government that are involved in assisting in the handling of emergency responses to incidents or assisting the states with handling emergency incidents. The NRT is co-chaired by the EPA and the U.S. Coast Guard.

National Terrorism Advisory System (NTAS): In January 2011, this system replaced the Department of Homeland Security's (DHS) color-coded advisory system as a method for communicating information about terrorist threats by providing timely, detailed information to the public, government agencies, first responders, airports and other transportation hubs, and the private sector. Under this system, DHS coordinates with other federal entities to issue formal, detailed alerts when the federal government receives information about a specific or credible terrorist threat. These alerts will include a clear statement that there is an "imminent threat" or "elevated threat." The alerts also will provide a concise summary of the potential threat, information about actions being taken to ensure public safety, and recommended steps individuals and communities, businesses and governments can take.

North American Emergency Response Guidebook (NAERG 2000): It was developed jointly by the U.S. Department of Transportation (DOT), Transport Canada (TC), and the Secretariat of Communications and Transportation of Mexico (SCT) for use by fire fighters, police, and other emergency services personnel who may be the first to arrive at the scene of a transportation incident involving a hazardous material. It is primarily a guide to aid first responders in

(1) quickly identifying the specific or generic classification of the material(s) involved in the incident, and (2) protecting themselves and the general public during this initial response phase of the incident. The NAERG 2000 is updated every three years.

Regional Response Team (RRT): The United States is divided into 10 federal regions and each has a response team made up of members from the same federal agencies that make up the NRT. The RRT interfaces with the states within its region and provides support to the state and local community emergency planning and response efforts.

Risk Analysis: A process or methodology used to evaluate the potential harm that may be caused by the inadvertent or purposeful release of a hazardous substance or material outside of its containment. The harm may be to humans, property, and/or the environment and determined by and ranked by the use of probabilities.

Risk Assessment (sometimes Risk Analysis): The process of determining the nature and scale of the losses or potential losses (due to catastrophes or disasters) that can be anticipated in particular areas during a specified time period. Risk assessment involves an analysis and combination of both theoretical and empirical data concerning the probabilities of known hazards of particular force or intensities occurring in each area (hazard mapping); and the losses (both physical and functional) expected to result from each element at risk in each area from the impact of each potential disaster hazard (vulnerability analysis and expected loss estimation).

Safety Officer: A member of the command staff at the incident or within an EOC responsible for monitoring and assessing safety hazards or unsafe situations at the scene of the emergency, and for developing measures for ensuring personnel safety. The safety officer may have assistants.

Sheltering in Place: This is the means of protecting the public by asking them to stay indoors in their homes and businesses until the danger of a harmful gas cloud or other hazard has been determined to have left the area. This determination of when the danger is over is to be made by local authorities in charge of the emergency response efforts.

Staging Area: The locations set up at an incident scene where resources can be placed while awaiting a tactical assignment. It is also the location where incident personnel and equipment are assigned on a three-minute available status or immediate deployment to an operational site within the disaster area.

State Emergency Operations Plan (also State Emergency Response Plan): A state plan that is designated specifically for state-level response to emergencies or major disasters and that sets forth actions to be taken by the state and local governments, including those for implementing federal disaster assistance.

Superfund Amendments and Reauthorization Act (SARA): This law required among other things the local emergency response planning efforts in every state through its Title III Emergency Planning and Community Right-to-Know Act of SARA.

Technical Specialists: Personnel with special skills who are activated only when needed. Technical specialists may be needed in the areas of fire behavior, water resources, environmental or medical concerns, resource use, industrial processes, hazardous chemicals, and training areas.

Termination Procedures: The part of the ICS in which staff and responders are involved in the preparation of records and documenting the on-scene management decisions, hazard concerns on the scene, and the critique results and discussions. Termination is divided into three phases: debriefing the response staff, post-incident analysis, and the critiquing of the emergency incident.

Terrorism: The calculated use of violence or the threat of violence to attain goals, which are political, religious, or ideological in nature. This can be done through intimidation, coercion, use of violence, or instilling fear. Terrorism includes a criminal act against persons or property that is intended to influence an audience beyond the immediate victims.

Unified Command: In ICS, unified command is a unified team effort that allows all agencies with responsibility for the incident, either geographical or functional, to manage an incident by establishing a common set of incident objectives and strategies. This is accomplished without losing or abdicating agency authority, responsibility, or accountability. Typically ICS is used in the early stages of an incident, but if it grows substantially larger, then the unified command is created at the top to manage the overall incident.

Vulnerability Analysis (or assessment): The process of estimating the vulnerability to potential disaster of specified elements at risk. For engineering purposes, vulnerability analysis involves the analysis of theoretical and empirical data concerning the effects of particular phenomena on particular types of structures. For more general socioeconomic purposes, it involves consideration of all significant elements in society, including physical, social, and economic considerations (both short- and long-term), and the extent to which essential services (and traditional and local coping mechanisms) are able to continue functioning.

Warm Zone: This zone represents an area of less potential for contaminant exposure to workers and is the zone that contains the decontamination area. The decontamination activity is located on the upwind and upgrade side and extends from the hot zone to the cold zone. This area may also be used to support the responders with miscellaneous equipment needs such as changing air bottles and replacing worn or damaged PPE. Exiting from the hot zone will be accomplished by going through the decontamination steps.

This Glossary was developed from Emergency Responder Guidelines, Office of Domestic Preparedness, Office of Justice, August 1, 2002 and updated by the National Safety Council, April 4, 2011.